PERMAFROST

PERMAFROST

Eva Baltasar

Translated from the Catalan by Julia Sanches

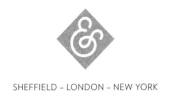

SHEFFIELD – LONDON – NEW YORK

This edition published in 2021 by And Other Stories
Sheffield – London – New York
www.andotherstories.org

Originally published in Catalan as *Permagel* by Club Editor in 2018.
© Club Editor and Eva Baltasar, 2018
All rights reserved by and controlled through Club Editor. This edition c/o SalmaiaLit,
Literary Agency.
Translation copyright © Julia Sanches, 2021

9 8 7 6 5 4 3 2 1

ISBN: 9781911508755
eBook ISBN: 9781911508748

Editors: Ana Fletcher & Stefan Tobler; Copy-editor: Larissa Melo Pienkowski; Proofreader:
Sarah Terry; Typesetter: Tetragon, London; Typefaces: Linotype Swift Neue and Verlag;
Cover Design: Anna Morrison. Printed and bound on acid-free, age-resistant Munken
Premium by CPI Limited, Croydon, UK.

A catalogue record for this book is available from the British Library.

And Other Stories gratefully acknowledge that our work is supported using public
funding by Arts Council England.

The translation of this book from Catalan has been partially funded by the Consortium
of the Institut Ramon Llull and partially supported by Acción Cultural Española, AC/E.

Supported using public funding by
**ARTS COUNCIL
ENGLAND**

GOBIERNO
DE ESPAÑA

AC/E
ACCIÓN CULTURAL
ESPAÑOLA

MIX
Paper from
responsible sources
FSC® C020471

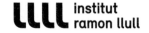
**institut
ramon llull**

CONTENTS

To poetry, for permitting it.

To be born is to be unhappy, he said, and as long
as we live we reproduce this unhappiness.

THOMAS BERNHARD, *THE LOSER*

1

It's nice, up here. Finally. That's the thing about heights: a hundred meters of vertical glass. The air is air at a higher degree of purity and so also seems harder, at times almost solid. There is a hovering smell of metal. A layer of noise hangs down below, soot-heavy and latent, like a fine, crisp eye of oil, a sort of shiny, black gift. Not even a bird flies by. They've got their own strata too, between us and our – let's say – gods. A livable void amid the top lines of a staff. Right now, I am and I am not. Maybe I'm just putting myself out there, declaring my presence, like a mildly annoying smudge on a lens, a dark cloud over this chill expanse. I take a breath and make it mine as it courses through my animate airways. Alive, I still give off a certain warmth and am probably oh-so-soft inside. On the outside, I'm softer than I might seem, as good as a pastry, a warm thing of varnished wax as alluring as an opening line. Every cell reproduces itself, independent of me, and in doing so reproduces me, fashioning me into a proper entity. If only all these microscopic parts of me stopped working, even for a second . . . Indivisible entities also deserve some time off, as do I, as do all the country's geniuses. Working with my cells, I am forced to adapt to them, to be like them, a small, anonymous goldfish inside this lovely glass enclosure. Beautifully decorative. Some restaurants place these sorts of fish on top of every table, inside tiny fishbowls. They're decorative, for sure. Soothing. They're very much alive, and yet some people use their homes as ashtrays. The poor little creatures perish, poisoned by the toxic chemicals in cigarette butts. But that's all they are, right? Ornaments. Frivolous lives.

The air is so pure! But not too humid, which is nice. Humidity has a nasty habit of penetrating the most vulnerable parts of our bodies. I can't stand it. I can't and don't know how to live with humidity, which slips into unsuspected corners inside me like icy, fatty lava and occupies unknown spaces, making me painfully aware of them. Some body parts, like oversized furniture, are practically impossible to manage. Apparently, they're not modular, and it would be too dangerous to remove them. Surely they must serve some purpose – someone must have stuck those pieces in there – but I just can't cope with them and the only way to escape their influence is to ignore them. To walk down the hallway with my eyes shut and not smash into their massive heft. Walking with my eyes shut – how charming! I hadn't thought about my eyes yet. Birds fly with their eyes open, and when they let themselves go, it's on solid currents of air. Suspended, and segmented, like marionettes. They allow themselves to look around. But if something were to fall . . . when a chick falls from its nest, for example, does it fall with its eyes open? Do birds even have eyelids? Or do they have the tear ducts of a frail granny, the kind that leak nonstop? To be fair, we're not talking about human eyelids. Maybe they're more like Japanese screens or those retractable shades on airplane windows, and maybe they trigger them in lightning bursts, just as fast as us or even faster. Now I wonder whether I'll open my eyes – or rather, if they'll be opened. Mine won't be just any fall. As in it won't be accidental. There will be an intention, an intended resolve, a pre-written command.

When the time comes, all I'll have to do is execute it. Eyes are pioneers; they probe the world and then the body responds. What sense is there in preparing the body for death seconds before it arrives? Like love, death catches the body. So let it be caught unawares.

2

"When you grow up, you'll understand," Mom never tired of saying. I must not have grown enough. Even though I made a conscious effort to drink all those glasses of milk, glasses as tall and wide as an animal's mouth, as big as my face, and that left a red tiara on my forehead where the rim of the glass had rested. They could hold so much milk that Mom always had to open another carton so she could fill the glass all the way up, practically to the brim. "Go on, pussycat, drink it all up," she'd say. "Stick out your little tongue and lap it all up like a good pussycat." Liters and liters of milk, and I was all white inside, coated with skins of milk inside, which clung like gooey, wet sheets to my walls and to the underside of my skin. Mom's tanks of milk wiped me out, they made me less human, even less of a girl. It was like I was half-girl, half-milk-tank, a sort of saturated vat. Once I was done drinking, I never dared to move; I could feel the milk dancing around inside my belly. No, not dancing, but sloshing recklessly like a pail of water on a brief and frenzied journey, then rushing down like water through the neighbor's bathroom pipes. Just like that, except inside me. I could feel the milk washing down what was left of my dinner, leaving everything with a fresh coat of paint – clean but gummy. The image was so striking that it forced me to stay very still, motionless, as my breath turned shallow. There was only one thing I could do to get through that time: read. I would sit in the only chair in my bedroom. My desk was pine with a white, childproof covering. "It's for your homework," Mom insisted once the carpenter was done assembling it. "No painting, no cutting, and don't even think of using the box cutter. Where is it, anyway? Shouldn't it be here? In the tin? With the scissors? Go find the box cutter and put it back where it belongs." With the scissors. And I don't understand it, I still don't, it makes no sense.

I've settled on an edge, I live on this edge and wait for the moment when I'll leave the edge, my temporary home. Temporary – like any home, in fact, or like a body. I'm not on medication. Chemicals are bridles that restrict you and slow you to a harmless pace. Chemicals mean early salvation; they ward off sin, or maybe they just teach us to label as sinful the exercise of freedom attained in times of peace – before death, of course. Mom self-medicates, Dad self-medicates, my sister didn't at first but now she does too, because she's grown-up and understood. Self-medication is a permanent temporary solution, like the low-watt bulb hanging in the hall. Twenty years with a dimly lit hall – how little it takes to become used to seeing so little. "We had halogen bulbs installed in the whole apartment and we forgot the hall!" Laughter. "And the best part is we didn't even realize until yesterday!" Twenty years had gone by. Twenty years of putting on lipstick three times a day, a hairbreadth away from the mirror, twenty years of fumbling blindly for the keys. I used to think it was normal – when you're a kid, your home life determines what's normal. And this normalcy shapes you. You grow up sheltered inside its patterns and take on its body, as does your brain, keen and malleable as clay. And then – though it takes years – the blindness cracks open under the force of a hammer striking over and over, but by then you're trapped inside the tight nucleus that has already taken 90 percent of all that was good in you to put some holes in. Get out now, if you can! And be happy while you're at it, like everybody else. Medication: quite the antidote. Not for me, though – best to keep moving wildly to the edge, and then decide. After a while, you'll find that the edge gives you room to live, vertical as ever, brushing up against the void. Not only can you live on it, but there are even different ways of growing there. If surviving is what it's all about, maybe resistance is the only way to live intensely. Now, on this edge, I feel alive, more alive than ever.

3

Safety precautions all over the place. More than people. More than rats. Precautions enacted without rhyme or reason. Safety precautions in the form of guardrails, bulletproof windows, no-trespassing signs, seat belts, helmets, alarm buttons, and blockades. Precautions that are active or passive, whatever. Knee pads, for example, or foam floor tiles, zippers, condoms, riot police, and football. Unemployment benefits and medication. Precautions that are subtle or obvious. Electromagnetic brakes, prisons, banners, social integration initiatives, scaffolding, valves, fireproof cladding, harnesses, and carabiners. And again, medication, hard hats, 2% milk. Medication, medication, and medication. A successful suicide, these days, is heroic. The world is full of unscrupulous people certified in first aid; they're everywhere, gray and unassuming like female pigeons but aggressive like mothers. They foil death with cardiac massages and careful Heimlich maneuvers. They're a pack of thieves. You can't even ram an olive pit down the wrong tube without them forcing you to spit it out, even if they break ribs or puncture lungs in the process. And there you are, covered in dry-martini puke, the olive pit hurled like a trophy at a corner of the room. I wouldn't mind dying in a corner. It should be possible to rent corners for dying in peace, without interference or self-activated oxygen tanks dropping down on you at the very last moment, corners where safety precautions guarantee – where they assure you – a proper death.

In reality, safety precautions are defenses against the outside world, the Supreme Torturer. The world unloads its toxicity into my core daily and assimilates me with its infiltration. But I can't allow it, I won't let myself partake. Lousy medication. Red and yellow pills lure me like flowers, a nectar for a bad life, a nourishing concoction. Who am I to refuse? My sister claims she is happy. Happy! That word had been gathering moss by the time I was born. When my sister says the word "happy" – "I'm very happy," she says – she bares her teeth. Her teeth gawk at me like eyes, yellowish like the whites of old people's eyes. And mind you, she quit smoking and drinking coffee before she hit her twenties. But rooibos and yoga are also addictive – they're acidifying, aging, and addictive. Healthy things kill you much more slowly. They begin by convincing you of their love and making you bow to their withering intensity. For decades, we're forced into a state of colorlessness, and in one of these decades we're inclined to reproduce. A stroke of genius! This reckless imposition of childhood can only be a side effect of medication. To enter life, you have to be as soft as stuffing, every new child swaddled from head to toe in the silk of fear – a castrating mother by nature, an unconditional cheerleader. The power of fear is in the sum of every small dream reduced to dust. Let's snort it, then – looks like that's the only way left to live. To conceal nudity by shutting it away in the shower, and peace at last. God bless sedation.

4

Railway tracks at an unmonitored location. Trains still bear witness to a certain metaphysics of habit – an observation that has nothing to do with schedules. Everything needs explaining. I only understood this on the day of my appointment at the unmonitored location. It was a thoroughly predictable straight line. Anybody else might have preferred a curve, but an incoming curve attracts too much attention – there's a subtle slowdown, an instant in which the body shifts its weight from one foot to the other, or perhaps gulps down saliva in an unusually conscious act. This straight line is perfect, and I am camouflaged by my surroundings. Mediterranean aridity mottled with sickly yet unyielding shrubs. The sound of something approaching, displacing cubic tons of suspended particles. I take a step forward. I sense the distantly booming mass, vibrations that could be insects and yet aren't, because insects are more elegantly metallic. The tracks shudder like rattlesnakes, and I take another step forward. My body is a parabola hungering for fear. The heart is large and conquers the mind. The train is now pure, barking mercury, a surging thing, a name. It's here now. It has reached me, its red tape, its finish line. No, not today. This train's too long, far too long, and it pitches my body violently backward. I decide not to yield. Like a shrub, I think. Deep roots support moments of courage such as this one. Still, the train is endless. There is too much steel for too long and maybe the body deserves a chance to speak after all – that thing about last words. Maybe I should keep my name, maybe I should die a conventional death with easily identifiable spoils and nice remains. The truth is, I never pictured myself caring about these sorts of details. I find myself caught up in a surprising metaphysics. If I were a believer, I might believe someone wanted me to reconsider things. How does it go again? "Thank God I'm an atheist."

5

It's a quarter past four in the morning and somebody has dialed my number. I'm not asleep, but my landline's disconnected and my cell phone is off. So what? It's how I stay human. And again at half past seven, ten to eight, eight to eight, and eight on the dot, followed by more failed attempts up until ten o'clock – all of it recorded in voice messages that I delete without listening to them. No doubt a consequence of ditching the meds. Considering I have no real reason to cause alarm, at ten I hook up both phones and answer the call. I activate chummy-voice mode. My sister horns in: "I'm pregnant again!" I dedicate my first thought to a forgotten mountain of spare tires. This news might be the incentive I need to clear out once and for fucking all. My second thought gets ready to endlessly dissect my sister's tone – the poor thing is wingless and naive and has no choice but to run, hefting her barefoot words. Her name is Cristina, and I still can't tell if Cristina is happy or upset. "Come again? I can't hear you." I ask questions and tell lies, tell lies and ask questions: that's how I roll. She says, without missing a beat: "I'm pregnant again! Two months in." She's happy – of course she's happy – and I'm a fool. "I'm so happy! We've been trying for ages." I have a nearly uncontrollable urge to bash in my skull with the phone. A terrible idea – phones are partial to murder by tumor, to long-distance deaths. "Congratulations,"

I say. "Are you happy?" she asks. I lie with an emphatic yes, so happy. "You're going to be an auntie again!" she exclaims. No matter how hard I try, I can't seem to detect a single emotion capable of shaking loose my interior bedrock of family relations. "That's great," I say. Then I talk. I rattle on for a minute straight, hoping to shortcut any attempts to plumb my emotional compost pile. "That's great really great oh my god it's so amazing to be an aunt twice over it's like being a full-fledged aunt like going from wearing a monocle to wearing a pair of glasses or from riding a tricycle to riding a bicycle I finally feel like I've got my life as an auntie under control hell you left me hanging for so long but suddenly here it is this little person who's decided to charge right into the wonderful business of living and it couldn't have hoped for better parents parents with stable jobs and a gorgeous house with a bedroom just for her or for him because of course two months in you don't have any way of knowing yet whether it'll be a boy or a girl though I don't actually know why I'm talking about it in the future since it's already a boy or a girl it already exists inside your belly oh it must be amazing to be pregnant and feel life growing inside you I'm sure this pregnancy will be as terrific as the first one and that everything will be great just great and it's so sweet of you to share this news with me you've made my morning this is the kind of news that makes a person feel like it's all worth it and besides when the family gets together for Christmas there won't be thirteen of us anymore which people say is bad luck but one more little girl or boy and that's just terrific." A colossal effort that leaves me dead tired. Seriously, this is the sort of behavior that drives people to medicate.

6

"Do you think I should marry him?" My aunt, some fifteen years ago. "It's just that sometimes on the metro, I can't help staring at other women's breasts. It's like they've been put there for me to stare at. And I wonder whether, maybe, before tying the knot, I should try and – " I'd always known the whole aunt thing didn't suit her. I let it slide, assuming she'd only asked because she knew I was gay. My mom still didn't know, but my aunt did. It had been six months since she'd let me crash at her bachelorette pad near my university. This saved me a three-hour daily commute, time I instead spent reading and meeting other lesbians. "I don't know," I began. Of course you shouldn't marry a dude when you'd just as well bury your face in some random woman's tits! "Maybe you should give it a shot. You know, just to make sure." "Maybe you're right. Lesbians are so ugly, though!" Thanks very much. She never caught on. There's nothing more blinding than blood. As expected, she decided it would be more sensible *not* to make sure. She didn't want to cheat on her "future husband," she said. So she married him, not realizing she had done something far worse: She'd committed the eminently literary act of turning her life into a big fat lie. Funny how sometimes the most wretched crimes are the easiest ones to carry off. After the wedding, she moved into a ground-level apartment in a residential neighborhood with a shared courtyard and neighbors who were reliable and self-contained, like supporting actors. All in all, it lent her a gleaming veneer of credibility. Oh, and she bought a family car too! "For whatever comes next," she said, as if the future specialized – exclusively – in knocking up women. I had the bachelorette pad all to myself. A top-floor apartment in the city center: perfection. I read day in and day out. Then came the internet boom, affording me unforeseen access to lesbians. Most of them weren't ugly, which resulted in a lot of sex – sex that was by and large good, but also sex that was so-so, and sex that was downright dire. Still, I couldn't seem to fall in love. I basically made friends, most of whom ended up as my lovers. Now and then, a lover would fall in love with me and I'd have the impression that life was staring me dead in the eye in its most unflattering wig. There's nothing worse than feeling like you belong entirely to someone else, having to hear that you're key to their happiness or unhappiness, reduced to a Lego block. Have we lost our minds? I also had several bizarre experiences, most of which fell on the days after the end of one of these relationships. Weirdly enough, I was never directly threatened, though I did participate in a couple self-mutilations, which was considerably worse. "Jesus, if you really want to slit open your wrists, just cut them vertically and get it over with already!" I sublet rooms to students so I could make ends meet without having to get a job. Women, exclusively: English women, American women, Brazilian women, German, Serbian, and Greek women. It was messy and sometimes fun, and there was the odd disturbance too. I'll never understand some women's obsession with drilling holes in the walls to hang their pictures. A whale-faced Basque girl set fire to the vent over the stove, and one night a gorgeous Brazilian with short legs ran off with the landline. But our dinner table conversations made it all worthwhile, and certain things made me feel really present, like the fact that sex was had in every room of the house and the bathroom was always occupied. Until one day, as if caught in an undertow, I graduated.

7

Real artists don't deal in the past. They make, in the Platonic sense of to create. People who don't know any better, like me, are the ones who end up stirring the great cauldron of history. Art history, in my case. At first I had been drawn to the fine arts, with the blind and limpid eagerness of youth. I really was anxious to create. The dream itself might have been enough to get me ahead – it was fresh as seashells, maybe even enriching. Except I harbored a deep insecurity that was fanned by my old-fashioned parents. "You can't even draw a face out of a six and a four," Mom used to say, exercising the frank concern with which she kept my self-confidence in a near-vegetative state. "Maybe you're right," I conceded at last. Doubt: the first chink in the permafrost. "Of course," she said. "Listen to us. Don't we always want what's best for you? Does anyone know you better than we do? You're too young to have any idea what you should or shouldn't do." I gave in out of exhaustion, but also out of irrational fear. Fear, domineering mother. Turns out it's practically impossible to wean off her tit.

It was like falling into a dead end that went on for five years. Knowledge bored into me, as though it thought it might find something of value inside. The day I graduated, I cried all evening long on the dining room sofa while the Serbian pianist from the bedroom off the entryway had me knock back ibuprofen and wine. I was mourning that whole contaminated terrain. "Now what?" I wailed. "I've lost five years of my life! It's too late to switch to a degree in fine arts." At twenty-three, it's too late for everything. Not until our forties do we realize there's still time. Maybe not for everything, but at least for everything that matters. After all, we've spent more than a decade trying to work out what's important. We got drunk, the Serbian and I. Her name was Jovana. She was forty-seven years old and a professional pianist. She was good but not good enough to make the top ten, and her musical talent just about kept her afloat. She was also strong, vital, and tremendously attractive, a sort of femme fatale who struggled to find love. One day, she dropped everything and moved to Barcelona. "I have a feeling this is where I'll meet my Antonio Banderas," she confessed when she sublet the room. Her whole life was folded into three Samsonite suitcases. The neighbor across the hall lent her an upright piano. I was stunned. Contrary to every expectation, the neighbors loved to hear her practice. They'd fallen for her, for the roundness of her body and for her personality, charming and formidable like a Burmese pagoda. I felt smaller and smaller by the day, next to her nothing but a frilly kitchen curtain. She was too much woman for me to even desire. I felt as disoriented as a war veteran struggling to adapt to civilian life. Like my life had been waylaid in a space that rippled with emptiness, and I had to keep in constant motion. I often felt queasy, like there was pressure on my lungs, a sort of preemptive anguish whose only relief was physical discomfort – period pain, for example. Month after month, I was plagued by a layer of lead that settled in my kidneys, by the growing need to move in fits like an insane person, by the roaring return of that familiar diarrhea, and by the enormous elephant foot that pressed down on my uterus over and over with irrevocable resolve. These episodes lasted from three to eight hours, and all of the prescription painkillers I took had no choice but to capitulate before the divine sovereignty of my body. There was nothing I could do. This torment always culminated in a sort of coma that left me prone at the very bottom of a deep slumber. The relief that followed was not unlike the end of a torture session, a feeling of absolute emptiness and levity. During these attacks, the queasiness would miraculously lift, though my suicidal tendencies became stronger than ever, as innocent as caga tió carols and just as cruel. I used to spend hours peering over the guardrail of the roof terrace. Eight stories, not bad. Shame there were so many cats scurrying around the ground floor. The thought of crushing one was agony. The neighbors who fed the cats tins of pâté as a way of calming their nerves deserved to be tossed in the Roman circus. Jovana insisted they weren't getting any, that they were starved of sex. "In Serbia, we make them into stew," she said. "What, you mean the cats?" "No, silly, sex-starved neighbors." "So, are there no sex-starved neighbors in Serbia?" "No, they all died in the war." War, a real godsend for cats. They say women prefer suicide by poison. But what kind? Cleaning products are too abrasive. A bleach cocktail? Forget it. In the fifties, you could sweet-talk your family doctor into giving you a prescription of barbiturates. Not anymore, though. Last time I went, the doctor suggested Bach Flower Remedies. I must not have been very convincing. Sex-starved neighbors, on the other hand, have medicine cabinets fit for nuclear bunkers. I know this because my granny is one of them. A lover of pigeons and cats, the woman has three dining-room cupboards chock-full of meds. I had a look inside one day: stacks upon stacks of pain management pills. How the hell do they do it? Are doctors sympathetic to cats? I'm not sure, but I suspect the sex-starved build up resistance. They're like cockroaches or water bugs, capable of scrubbing their faces in sizzling hot oil.

8

"Why not work as an au pair for a year?" I'm not sure who said this, but I know it wasn't Mom because I wouldn't have listened to her. Au pairing? Wasn't that for girls without the brains to get into university? I already had a degree! "Yeah, a degree in sitting on the couch all day twiddling your thumbs." Untrue. I'm not sure who said that, but I remember thinking it was a lie. Yes, I sat on the sofa all day, but I was reading. For a while I was into biographies, the fatter the better. Great personalities are always giving copious pages of themselves: de Beauvoir, Raffaello, Mallarmé, von Bingen, Łempicka, Gentileschi, Kokoschka, Kahlo, Lessing, Van Gogh, Foucault, Cassatt, Claudel, Weil, Cézanne, Napoleon. The pleasure I felt in sinking my waking hours into the lives of other people – full and perfect lives, bookended by two dates worthy of celebration – was indescribable. Spending my days like that was the best I could aspire to, the closest I could get to neither coming to an end nor arriving at a beginning. I was happy enough just subletting the apartment's three spare bedrooms. Sure, they were on the small side, but they were just right for one person. Futon mattresses, desks, closets. Colorful bedsheets, original lamps, and a hideous terrazzo floor covered wall to wall in a sixteen-millimeter-thick rug. God bless IKEA. The apartment was relatively inexpensive and the atmosphere laid-back, so the rooms never went empty.

I kept that scheme going for three years – the best three years of my life. What I wanted was to live effortlessly, like a little worm-eaten branch that floats downstream with no ambition other than to drift along, bowing to every change in direction and embracing its weathering. It was also a time of solitary sex. I was tired of sifting through the various lesbian cliques of Barcelona, worn out from sharing flesh. That's when it happened, just when I seemed to have reached peak happiness: a midafternoon phone call. Midafternoon phone calls are the worst kind of phone call. There's something passionate about the catastrophe of a midnight phone call, an attempt on life by jump-starting the heart. We should all be on the receiving end of at least one midnight call a month, so that we can carry on living at another level of intensity. A midafternoon call, on the other hand, is a torpedo: "Hello?" "It's your aunt. I need the apartment." I had a clear image of the guillotine dropping and my head bouncing on the floor like a furry ball, then rolling away until it vanished beneath the sofa. Shit. "No problem. When?" "There's no rush. We can meet for the keys once you find a place." Apparently, there was a rush. "Are you splitting up?" If so, at least there would be hope for somebody. "No, we want to buy a house. We're selling the apartment." Well, look at that. My aunt had decided to boldly probe the uncharted depths of her lie. "That's great," I said. By evening, the conviction that I was being wrongfully discharged had taken root inside me. The injustice of it lodged in my throat in the shape of a wood egg. "What now?" I asked myself over and over. Should I find a room to rent? My degree wasn't worth a damn, and I had no income to speak of. Maybe I could life-model at the Facultat de Belles Arts, I thought, and wondered if the students would be willing to sketch me lounging naked on a sofa as I read. I could think of no other way to maintain my lifestyle – an irrational idea that was nonetheless painfully real. For a few minutes, it felt like the only solution. Either that or throw myself off the balcony. Now of all times, when it had been years since I'd given it any serious thought. Knowing my luck, I'd end up squashing a cat. Whoever came across my body would instead find two, innards in a knot like a snake nest. No, that wouldn't do at all.

Suddenly, everything became clear to me. I called Jovana. We weren't living together anymore. She was shacked up with Antonio Banderas in a second-floor apartment at Ronda Sant Pere, or at least that's what she'd told me. "I'm fucked," I said the second she picked up. "You?" "Yeah, my aunt's kicking me out. I'm a family refugee." I felt sorry for myself. "She's doing you a massive favor." Bullshit. "You'll thank her in a few years. You can stay with us if you want. We've got plenty of room." "No, thanks. I've always been a bit scared of Antonio Banderas." "Aren't you a lesbian?" "Yeah, but guys who sound like cats frighten me." "What is it with you and cats?" "I don't know. They give me the creeps." "Why not work as an au pair for a year?" Now I remember. It was Jovana who said it. Also the thing about having "a degree in sitting on the couch all day twiddling your thumbs." "What can I say, I like reading," I said. "So go work as an au pair. You can read all day long." Jovana assured me that all I would have to do was take the kids to school, and some light dusting. I might even be given a small salary. Maybe, I thought. Sure, maybe. Doubt: the rift through which the world's heat slips in, a brazen violation of the permafrost.

9

Cardrona, Scotland. I had always thought the world's smallest towns sat deserted at the tops of tall mountain ranges. I was wrong. Cardrona is microscopic, a cluster of modest houses in an infinite golf course, like the mound of dirt that signals an anthill in a bare field. Despite what movies would have you believe, small towns are boring. It's just about impossible to meet anyone interesting. My host family's house has two floors and a garden rendered useless by fine, unrelenting rain. What matters is that two children live here, a boy and a girl. They're pale, dumpy, and soft. Their mother, like all respectable Scottish mothers, is named Fiona. Fiona works in sales for a pharmaceutical company, so she spends a lot of the year traveling. Their father isn't in the picture. Jovana was right, all I do is take the kids to school and some light dusting with the duster. The rest of the time, I read in my room. In it is a single bed with a solid wooden headboard and a patchwork quilt that's hideous but appropriate. There's also a small desk on top of which sat an empty picture frame when I first arrived. The sight of it made me think of Mom, so now it lives in the drawer. The window is large and U-shaped. The scenery is breathtaking, like a tinted seascape. Outside are fields as far as the eye can see, carpeted in emerald hay that heaves like a lung. If I stare at them long enough, I begin to feel an unsettling lack of salinity. By the window, inlaid beneath the hollow of the U, is a seat with floral upholstery. When I sit on it, I feel like Scarlett O'Hara. But it's a good refuge from the excessive heating. I start a new book every two days, and within a week have already worked my way through the ones I brought with me. My initial, perfectly realistic estimate had been of a month. Cardrona surpasses my every expectation. I soon find myself wishing the kids would never grow up. All I want is to be a lifelong au pair, and I have curious impulses, like the urge to withhold their food. Frail children physically remain children for longer, though some abuse has also been known to accelerate emotional maturity. My chances of success are slim, but it's worth a shot. I spend hours daydreaming about accidents that involve the staircase, and about the possibility of one of the siblings becoming paralyzed. Maybe the girl. A man who is crippled is statistically more likely to find a partner than a woman in the same situation. I'm sure that if the girl were to become paralyzed, Fiona wouldn't hesitate to hire a competent au pair on an indefinite basis.

These thoughts are so soothing I don't need to act on them, so I leave them alone and order a copy of *A History of World Art* online. Ten just-like-new secondhand volumes for under four hundred euros, an investment that translates into six months of uninterrupted pleasure. Long before I'm done reading, I am assaulted by the delirious notion that I wasted my time at university. I can't get my mind off fine arts, the soul of the dead matter in which I received my degree. This realization gives way to a series of symptoms: a stabbing pang in the chest; difficulty eating and drinking; another kind of pain that is slippery rather than stabbing and radiates from its epicenter in my uterus to every extremity of my body like a weighty, ravenous sorrow. It dawns on me that this must be like the pain that follows an abortion, the residual sadness of a life unlived, clinging clawlike to life. At night, I experience intense feelings of despair and spend my waking hours morbidly engrossed in a train of thought titled "Too Late for Fine Arts." Studying has always been a powerful distraction, like being temporarily stranded at a gas station. After all, moments like these are moments of death lost to themselves. The journey later resumes, and life converges with it, concentrated in isolated capsules of movement.

I lose weight without trying. The art books prove so painful I move on to philosophy. Philosophers are indeed orderly people. Germans, in particular, are second to none, complex yet orderly. The French, however, evoke the wonder felt on arriving home after a loved one has tidied up, watered the plants, and gone away again, leaving behind them a boundless sense of freedom. The philosophy texts last twice as long. Philosophy, an excellent investment! I spend way too much time playing Scarlett O'Hara at the window. It wouldn't surprise me if Mammy were to walk into my room at the crack of dawn with a corset in her arms, the scent of coffee and bacon wafting in behind her. It must be wonderful to surrender to the hands of a meaty Mammy, as comforting as an overflowing pantry in late fall. But I'm alone; I am fifty-two kilos of loneliness and lamentation, a real treasure.

I start hating the color green. Staring out the window has the same effect on me as drinking the tap water in India: nausea and near-constant headaches. Too much time at the window ends inevitably in long sessions on the toilet. But the order of this nausea is a little different; hungry for flesh, it expels the self and takes pleasure in wringing the juices from my body. Meanwhile, the self languishes in a peculiar bubble that bobs, sentimental and hollow. Scottish green is anomalous, flat and rich like an exercise in Fauvism. Cézanne would have found it a nightmare. Cézanne could never have been Scottish. This green is indulgent and verges on offensive. It visually assaults me like Matisse's red table, except without the ensuing peace and childlike calm. It annoys me to have my deep-seated love for Matisse compromised by an unsettling coat of green. Green permeates my body like a horse shot; it rises like a suffocating tide, floods every cavity, and colonizes the most fertile parts of my ego. I have the frightening urge to end this relentless unease by leaping out of the window. A lousy idea – the window isn't far enough from the ground. A death on damp garden tiles doesn't really appeal to me. I can't stomach the thought of a slug accidentally trailing its miserable life over my miserable death, or of using my dying breath to gnaw on fragments of words as leftover thoughts gush down my forehead in plain sight and my eyes take on the sympathetic look of a server at a late-night bar. A week later, I go home.

10

I'm home. Home is actually the guest room of my sister's rental apartment. The bedroom is small and plain, like a prison cell. There is a mattress on the floor, a plastic orange coatrack behind the door, and a wardrobe full of junk. I kill hours of insomnia rifling through the contents of the closet. Old clothes and white hotel towels, plus a couple of my sister's photo albums. It's weird to see her with friends I've never met. Sisters lead identical lives until one of them grows up, and then the other begins to do things in secret – above all, meeting new people to fill the hole her sister has left.

I study these photos. In twenty or so, my sister is with a boy who is pale and blond, golden-blond like a lioness. In thirteen, they are apart, and in the other seven, they're hugging. The pale boy with lioness-blond hair – with reddish eye rims and a nose as tense as a gymnast's ass – is most likely Scandinavian. I recall that my sister went to Denmark on her year abroad. Maybe he was a Danish fling. The boy looks at my sister, who looks at the camera. The fact that I know so little about my sister's life triggers a fledgling resentment. I stifle the feeling, remembering she had lived her life just as I had: at the margins of our family. I wonder why. There must be a reason. Both of us had craved intensity and if we'd kept on living with our family, it would've been diluted. Family, a first-rate solvent! You can't possibly reach the epicenter by their side. Some individuals can only grow as amputations. I picture my parents as the head of an octopus and my sister and me as its rambling tentacles – purple, roseate cartilage. But she really is sick. She's an ectoparasitic organism driven to couple with a male counterpart to keep her lie in balance. But she laughs, and much more than I do. In photos, she looks present, so fucking present. Not me, I always look like I've been superimposed. As if someone more childish yet far more powerful than any of us had a collection of paper-doll mes in various positions and decided to cut along my dotted outlines before pasting me into photos of other people, who would later insist that they knew me. That's me: the stranger everyone knows by sight, the one who appears fake beneath her layer of low and carefully mown grass. I have a decent covering, watertight like a ship's hull. It's true: This icy firmness stores a world that is habitable, yet dormant.

11

I only found work years later. Proper work, I mean, something in line with what I'd studied. Those five years would have been wasted otherwise. I don't think Mom could have coped. They'd poured so much money into me. "We put in so much effort! And went through so much hardship! One summer, we couldn't go away on vacation because your university fees went up. And, of course, you studied so hard. You were full of promise!" This all happened before the Bologna Process, but it's always been one of my family's greatest hits, our/their best record. "The summer we couldn't go on holiday because you needed braces." "I still remember that summer when we couldn't get away because your glasses broke and you needed a new pair." "And what about that summer when we didn't move house so that you could take a two-week intensive tennis course?" "And that year we bent over backward to get you a math tutor? We were so shocked! A clever girl like you failing math in her first year of high school. We may have lost the down payment on the caravan, but it was worth it. At least you passed math once September came around. There was a heat wave that summer too. It would've been lovely and cool in Switzerland. But we've always put kids first under our roof. Isn't that right, dear?" Isn't it right that when Mom goes on like this all you can think about is knives?

They hired me on a Monday, three months after my first article. For the first time, I felt colorless – a dreadful muddle of various hues, an unthinkably grim and grayish green. My skin was like a mollusk shell, my body parched, my muscles fibrous like esparto grass – and inside I smelled of a parking lot. In the evening, I received a congratulatory phone call. "We knew you'd figure things out eventually." It was Mom, the family spokesperson. "Thank you." "People-like-you need time." People like me. "But you found your way in the end. With everything you've put me and your dad through." I don't think I put Dad through anything, but I guess Mom thought of Dad as an extension of herself, a sort of infra-ego that formed an indivisible part of her. "Don't be so dramatic, Mom." These words usually gave her wings and allowed me to remain quiet. "But it's true! It's true. Your-dad-and-I went through tough times when you were younger, didn't we? Think about it, you're only just figuring things out at forty!" Tough times, figuring things out . . . Mom's basic vocabulary. "If you say so," I said. "Of course I say so. But don't think I'm trying to steal your thunder. Okay? Your-dad-and-I have read all three of your articles and they're outstanding. I don't understand why you didn't do this earlier. And to think you wasted the best years of your life loafing around this God-given Earth without ever doing much at all. Your teachers always said so. They were already saying so in primary school – she's full of promise, your daughter. It looked like you weren't amounting to anything, and I nearly went and complained. But look, you've finally found your focus. And your-dad-and-I are so proud, we're just so proud of you." It's worth noting that my-dad-and-her have never been proud of me or my sister. All my dad needs is to know we are happy-and-healthy. "Are you happy and healthy?" he asks when Mom hands over the phone so she-can-give-the-tortillaa-quick-flip. What matters to Mom, on the other hand, is our "occupation." And I don't just mean our profession, but all our labels, filing drawers filled with cards scribbled on in good Latin, like in the Natural History Museum. My sister, for example, has degrees in pharmacy and physical therapy. She's doubly qualified. According to Mom's values scale, this is very, very good. She's also married – she is the wife-of – and her husband is an engineer, for which she receives bonus points. She has a daughter and another boy/girl on the way, which means she is also the mother-of. She works part-time at a pharmacy in town. As far as I'm concerned, that's a shitty gig for two degrees, but Mom is over-the-moon. Not proud: over-the-moon. My sister can't work as a physical therapist because touching bodies makes her queasy. I understand this perfectly because I'm the same. The thought of touching another body makes me want to gag, unless it's during sex. The fact that my sister studied physical therapy baffles me.

The thing is that Mom saves her pride for herself. This way, she can apply the highlights from her mental vault to her own virtues. For example, Mom is proud of the fact that she never puts on an ounce of weight over Christmas, and also of her ever-immaculate apartment. She has a Peruvian woman come over three times a week to sweep, dust, deep-clean the bathroom, and mop. The sofa is vacuumed and the windows washed once a week. The kitchen cupboards are seen to every fifteen days and the oven and fridge once a month. Before the Peruvian woman there was an Ecuadorian woman, but she was building a house in her home country and left the moment she made the last payment. "A house with a little kiosk attached, now isn't that clever?" Mom said. "And to think we need all sorts of things to be happy. You should've seen María's face the day she told me she was going back to Ecuador. She has two kids over there. She was pure happiness. She was over-the-moon about her little kiosk house." If Mom were put in charge of a kiosk house, she'd fall into a depression so deep it would make the Great Crash look like a weekend getaway to the Costa Brava. As far as my current occupation goes, I think Mom is pleased – pleased that she has, at long last, put me in a box. Her eldest girl had come out slippery as an eel, but she's finally "found her focus." Honestly, if this is what focus means, I'm going to need some industrial-strength drugs to keep my head quiet and still in its cage.

12

"Épouse-moi!" Though I've had fabulous lovers, they're never so fabulous as the day I leave them. "Marry me," Veronika said again. She looked stunning. She was big, larger than me by at least three dress sizes – a Belgian with the bearing of a Viking, educated at the best universities in Flanders and the United States. Her flesh was firm and plentiful and her breasts soft and round as water balloons. She had thick, silken hair that reminded me of the surreal bundles of fiber optics that a technician had once threaded through the façade of my Barcelona apartment. Her eyes were impressive, an intricate glass mosaic that stared into mine, pulsing like a fetus and inexplicable as a miracle, when she came beneath me. We both loved chocolate. We used to buy Godiva bonbons, shut ourselves up in her apartment, and eat them in bed, letting the chocolate melt over our skin. Food play is a weakness of mine. She was seven years my senior and held some sort of managerial position at C&A. We'd met by chance, and if there's one thing I believe in, it's chance. Despite the Herculean efforts of new religions to deny it, chance continues to exist. I had moved to Brussels three months earlier and was renting a room from a woman in her late sixties. Her name was Brigitte and she wore dentures. Brigitte had a huge, shaggy, ancient black dog that slept in my room on a makeshift bed on a carpet of its own furballs. The dog's name was Taps. My room was the largest in the house, and it had everything: a double bed with a lumpy mattress, a faded yet comfortable sofa, a run-down wardrobe, an old desk, a fine chest of drawers, a sound system, and a TV. It was a centrally located, decently priced mini-studio. Brigitte represented what I imagined my future would have looked like if my aunt hadn't put me out on the street: a lifetime pensioner with an autistic dog as her only companion. She was very friendly. "Que fait une fille comme vous à Bruxelles?" I explained that I had just graduated from university and there were no jobs in my home country. The truth was I hadn't bothered to look. Desperate to get out of Barcelona, and with enough money in my pocket for six or seven months of inexpensive rent, I decided to travel. I'd chosen Brussels because a city whose symbol is a little boy pissing was a city I knew I would like. I didn't tell my parents until a few weeks after moving – a policy of fait accompli, a matter of survival. My savings began to dwindle. A couple of months later, I published an ad in a magazine – "Spanish teacher," it read – and quickly forgot about it. A man called me to hold what some might consider a fishy conversation. The voice on the other end sounded British and claimed to run a language school. He was in urgent need of a Spanish teacher and scheduled a meeting with me in a neighborhood on the outskirts of town. I consulted Brigitte, who confirmed that the neighborhood was as fishy-sounding as the phone call.

On the morning of the interview, I left a note on the oilcloth on the kitchen table, where I knew Brigitte would find it, with the school's address and instructions to call Interpol if I wasn't home within twenty-four hours. I was hesitant at first, but then it dawned on me that risking life and freedom for money was actually common practice, and at the very last minute, I decided to take Taps with me. An excellent plan. He didn't make me feel any safer, but having something other than myself to worry about made it harder for me to turn back. It was a long metro ride and Taps sat in my lap, which quickly went numb. Then a dead-legged transfer, hobbling like a blind woman with her seeing-eye dog. The next car was mostly empty. I noticed that for every station there seemed to be a prototypical rider. Sometimes, the same prototype spanned two or three stops. At other times, there were multiple prototypes per station. Yet they gradually gained definition. By the last stop, I felt completely out of place. As I walked out of the car, a teenager strung out on drugs made way for me. God bless Belgians! Friendliest Europeans I know. While I contemplated what exit to take, a tired woman weighed down by Colruyt bags came toward me. The bags under her eyes looked even heavier than her Wednesday shopping. Taps was restless, snuffling left and right in that obsessive way dogs have of sniffing out other animals' piss. I decided to let myself be led by his instincts, and we made it onto the street. There, I followed directions scribbled on a Post-it that fit into the palm of my hand. I had no trouble finding the address.

The building could have been worse. I rang the bell and the door opened as if somebody upstairs had been waiting for me with their finger on the buzzer. This set me on edge. They hadn't even asked for my name. I was about to turn around and leave when Taps nudged the door open with his wet snout and dragged me in. The lobby was passable. Traces of urine drowned out by liters and liters of bleach hung in the air, but there was an elevator and a couple of decent-looking strollers parked under the letterboxes. I pivoted toward the staircase. I was in no mood to shut myself in a cage with an animal, even if the animal in question was Taps, who I shared a room with every night. On the third floor, a young-looking British guy stood leaning against the door frame to his apartment, waiting for me. He ushered me into a large, empty space with no visible furniture. The Brit was bald and friendly and he smiled at us – at Taps and me in turn – twice. It dawned on me that the apartment might be a front, that in a back room somewhere, a hoard of pretty girls was possibly gagged and bound, hands and feet tied together with one long, improbably knotted rope. My mouth went dry. What would become of me? I wasn't even pretty! A thousand thoughts formed and evaporated like spray, like lattice flashes of night, fluctuations on a spectrometer. The British guy led us into an office, where I was surprised to see a table, office chairs, and a long bookcase full of textbooks. The sudden drop in my adrenaline made me dizzy, so I sat down. The British guy then explained his business to me. He had teachers of "every language" working for him. His clients were large companies, and he arranged private classes for their managers at their homes on a predetermined schedule. He could pay me forty-five euros an hour. Forty-five euros an hour! And his profit margins were probably still high. I couldn't believe it, but even so, I took the job and gave the clever Brit my account number, knowing full well I shouldn't. In exchange, he handed me his business card, Spanish textbooks 1, 2, and 3, and a timetable. I also signed a contract of unclear legality. Honestly, I couldn't have cared less. We said goodbye and he told me he would call once he'd arranged classes with my first client. I hurried out, Taps panting behind me as though he had asthma. As I sat on the metro, I realized my legs were shaking – but I was happy! Like I'd been sent away to summer camp while my friends were all stuck in iron lungs, a strange kind of happiness that comes from narrowly escaping disaster. I returned Taps to his owner in adequate condition and spent lunch leafing through the textbooks.

My phone rang around midafternoon. When work-related, midafternoon phone calls are by and large inoffensive. It was the great British entrepreneur, *my boss*, passing on contact details for my first student. Her name was Veronika Goossens and she was a manager at C&A. She lived in an apartment in the city center and had no knowledge of Spanish. Her employer had requested an intensive course of seven-and-a-half hours a week, Monday to Friday, six to seven-thirty in the evening, hours that didn't suit Brussels natives because they coincided with their near-mandatory leisure time. But I was an immigrant, on top of which I often found leisure tedious. In any case, I spent most of it reading, and it didn't matter to me when I read. I found Veronika's address on the map and gave myself a once-over in the mirror. I'd need to do something about my appearance or risk not being let off at her metro stop – a minor prototype issue easily solved with a lightning-fast trip to the mall. I spent the next morning "shopping" and arrived home with half a new wardrobe. It wasn't quite my style, but it would do: elegantly sober with minimal froufrou. I purposefully avoided C&A. At five to six in the evening, I rang the bell of a spectacular house on a street perpendicular to Grand Place. It wasn't far from where I lived, but there was no comparison. An exquisite woman answered the door. In under two seconds, I recovered my sex drive, which had lain forgotten in the double-bottom of a suitcase kept under a protuberance-plagued mattress. Some women make me feel wholly lesbian. It's not that I've never been attracted to men, it's just that there are women with whom I'm a lesbian only to a point. The lesbian is pitted against a whole series of simultaneous roles, as in a clash of intensi-ties. My ego is permanently populated by protected tenants: the daughter, the sister, the friend, the former university student, the neighbor, the reader, the auntie, the landlady, the client, the user, the confident one and her opposite, etc. Every one of these scrappy women coexists with and rivals the lesbian. But faced with Veronika, the lesbian sounded her ear-piercing cry for so long and at such a volume that I had to force the Spanish teacher to speak up. And yet I wasn't the one who spoke; the lesbian had subdued my innermost self and I was completely compliant. She was the one making my other voices speak and they were small, docile puppets in her hands. "Bonsoir. Je suis la professeur d'espagnol." She smiled. A burst of pale pink in her grin revealed teeth as perfect as polished icicles. "Bonsoir. Je suis Veronika. Enchantée." She bent over ever so slightly and gave me three kisses. Our cheeks hardly touched, but I felt her makeup graze the down on my face, keen as sensors. She led me into the living room. The apartment was a refurbished unit in a hundred-year-old building, and everything had the romantic look of the old-but-new. Every design was simple, with the exception of a piece of restored furniture that, though unexpected, blended in like an attractive and spirited orphan. Every surface seemed smooth and flat. There wasn't a single handle on the furniture, whose edges were polished but never overly rounded. The space flowed in a steady arrangement of white orchids. In fact, there was a lot of white and gray all around. In her too; she exuded the utmost tidiness. Her skin was lily-white and her blazer dark gray. An ivory sweater grasped her neck like a hand, delivering up a face whose focus was a pair of high and wide-set eyes, warm and strangely potent islets of light. A rectangular clip of mother-of-pearl held her hair in a low ponytail, every single strand of it, as if they'd each been collected and counted before being gathered up, as if they were all the same size, even the obnoxious fuzz around the temples, which I'd had since breastfeeding age. We sat at the dining-room table and she offered me a drink. We agreed that classes would be conducted in Spanish and any queries handled in English because my French wasn't up to the task. The lesbian stepped back and let me teach an adequate lesson, despite being repeatedly distracted by her hands. I fucking love women's hands. Delicate skin pulled thin like a membrane of constellations, tapered fingers, and the almost lyrical movement of joints. Veronika wore her nails short and coated in clear nail varnish. Short, the way I like them. I had this thought dozens of times. Short, the way I like them. Short, the way I like them. The one repeating this was actually my cunt, unrepentant thinker. An hour and a half later we said goodbye, until tomorrow. Veronika had to learn as much Spanish as she could in six months because she was being sent to Central and South America on temporary positions. C&A was conquering new horizons.

13

Fucking cell phone. Every time it rings, I think: I'll take it down with me. Take my contacts down too while I'm at it. It's my sister. "Hello?" "Hi, honey!" Mom? "It's a girl! She's here! Your little niece has come into the world. Let me put your sister on." Being the bearer of important news: the only climax Mom has ever known.

14

I've just scrubbed the tub. Sitting in it was so gross I had to scrape orange, crab-shaped glue off the bottom, leaving behind marks edged in black mold that refused to come out. I look it up online and go to the supermarket for steel scouring pads and bleach. Scrub-a-dub-dub. After fifteen minutes, the mold has retreated, but the crab silhouettes are still there, apparently burnt into the ceramic. It's odd – astonishing, even – what the passage of time does to the adhesive properties of certain glues. Glue was probably more aggressive twenty years ago than it is today. Everything was more aggressive twenty years ago; there were even heavy metals in baby bottles. This must be why boomer babies are such a remarkable generation, drugged from the cradle. I fill the bathtub all the way with lukewarm water and immediately realize I've made a mistake. I should shower first. I lather my head and body, rinse, wring my hair, and towel-dry my conscience. I start over, for real this time. In movies, before going through with it, women paint their lips and nails bright red. It's always seemed like a quaint touch to me. Do they really think they'll still look good three hours later, or the next day, or in two weeks' time? I'm in no mood for romance – I'm in a hurry. This time, it's for real. I use a square of toilet paper to collect a tangle of hair from the bathtub drain, toss it in the bowl, and flush. Even though it's mine, that soft cluster of fur sitting in a hole dotted with smaller holes grosses me out. I fill the tub all the way again with lukewarm water and take the candles out of the Schlecker grocery bag. They're decent enough candles, square with three wicks each and scents like Japanese cherry blossom or Fiji water lotus. I also take out the Gillette razors, half a dozen plus two freebies, all spanking new. I've never used one. Never even touched one, now that I think of it. The razors come in an indestructible plastic bag that I have to tear open with nail clippers. I leave them on the toilet lid, along with the candles. They look funny sitting there next to each other, like old letterpress T's. For some reason, I think of Virginia Woolf. Maybe because of her husband, who ran a press in their town. But Virginia Woolf had it better. The Ouse was clean, unlike the rivers here, which are flat-out polluted, their banks patrolled by sports nuts. I don't know why I didn't think to grab a book. Would I even be able to read? Would I have the time? I start to feel annoyed. I haven't planned things out as well as I thought I had. My elbow grazes the shower curtain – a cheerful-looking curtain riddled with butterflies of all colors. Shit. I've just spotted a patch of mold on the bottom edge, an impressive fungal network that spreads upward from the seam. I wonder if the curtain should hang inside or outside the bathtub. From up close, it's even grosser than the crab-shaped mold. I don't need it. I take down the metal rod and roll up the curtain. There. I decide to put it in the sunroom. It can't stay here. There isn't space for it in the bathroom. Besides, part of me still wants the site of my last moments to be an attractive one – or, if not attractive, at least tidy. I look like a demented soldier as I rush naked down the hallway with my blunt spear and flimsy butterfly shield. I go back. The bathroom looks better without the curtain. And without the rod. Bare rods are bleak, and it's a good thing I took it down. I'm not asking for much. Just a dignified death, a death from blood loss. They say it's like falling asleep. I have to pee. People on death row always have to pee. But I'm not on death row. If I don't go now, will piss trickle out of me after I die? I guess the body's sphincters must relax, especially in hot water. What about anal sphincters? I don't think so, but there's no reason to believe some sphincters do and others don't. I'd really hate it if my sphincters were to relax after I died. I decide to pee. I do it in the bidet, because the toilet is occupied by candles and Gillette razors. Should I give myself an enema? Mom used to take suppositories for number twos, but only when she felt like she had to go. I don't have to go, and I don't have suppositories. What I do have are five blank cartridges my dad gave me when I was little – a souvenir from his time in the military. And maybe they'd do the trick, even if they don't come out afterward, even if they stay inside me, and even if, for whatever reason, they have to do an autopsy. It would be tough on the coroner. I'm scared. My fear has thoughts, possessive thoughts that will have to be eliminated. I wash my cunt with a spurt of water and dry myself with a hand towel. I empty the corners of the bathtub of shampoo bottles, bodywash, conditioner, intimate wash, moisturizer, almond oil (I think of cyanide), and drop everything in the bidet. I grab the candles. Too big – they slip and fall in the water, getting everything wet. Fuck. Dozens of droplets turn almost instantly cold on my skin. Now I have goosebumps. No, no, no. This is not the state of mind I need to be in. I glance at the Gillette razors, which look harmless even though I know they aren't. I grab a razor and slice my wrist. Vertically. Without looking. I stop. I feel nothing. Though they say that cutting your veins is painless. I look down at my wrist. Nothing. I look at the razor. I study the razor. Gillette piece of shit – there's a see-through cap on the blade. I have no idea what the hell a Gillette razor should look like, but this thing in my hands is just a harmless fucking epilator.

15

"What's it like with a woman?" My sister, at a quarter to midnight. We're sitting in her small, adorable living room. This was just after she ended things with some boyfriend, and I had no choice but to be there for her. A considerate sister is like an information leaflet for contraceptives, with a list of contraindications and side effects as dangerous as a Gorgon. At eleven, I decided to order Chinese food. "Almond chicken, sweet-and-sour prawns, beef noodles, and fried rice." I always choose the same thing to spare myself having to reread those dismal menus. "Oh! And steamed buns." "Any drinks?" the Chinese man asks. What do I know. "Cris, what do you want to drink?" My sister gestures impotently from behind a barricade of tissues. She is at the pinnacle of self-pity, a place incompatible with speech. "A Coke and a Nestea," I hazard. He has me repeat the address three times. I hang up, walk to the sofa, and start collecting wads of tissues. The cold touch of the moist tissues is shockingly unpleasant. It troubles me that a certain kind of sadness can generate so much garbage. I take the empty box from the end table and in its place set down a roll of toilet paper that smells like talcum powder and is embossed with puppies – a temporary solution. "Be right back," I say. I pull on a jacket, bundle myself up in a scarf, and grab the keys and some money. My sister's tastes do not mesh with the kind of tissues they sell at the Pakistani corner store, so I walk down Gran de Gràcia toward Diagonal. I trot. My sister is functionally impaired and the last thing I need is for the Chinese takeout to reach the apartment before I do. I enter Opencor, which is at once pleasant and unsettling. It's always nice to go somewhere this late at night and find everything neat and tidy, all the clerks as fresh as baguettes. It inspires a sense of safety, as well as a certain unease on account of the two or three customers shuffling around in their magnetic fields of loneliness. I try not to make eye contact and grab three Ágatha Ruiz de la Prada tissue boxes, dainty and colorful as baubles. Hearts, flowers, kisses. They're so off-putting I'm sure my sister will like them. I head to the wine section and select two bottles of red based on the label. "Enuc del Priorat," one of them says. Maybe the closeness to "eunuch" will exert a subliminal influence on my sister and help her trivialize her relationship with the ex-boyfriend. An unfortunate purchase that will nonetheless help me close in on my goal: to escape my sister's toxic gravitational pull as quickly as humanly possible. At the cash register, I grab a packet of gum for "60 minutes of freshness." Chewing gum makes me gassy, but I read somewhere that it improves focus, which I'll need heaps of tonight so that I don't forget my lines. Thirty euros altogether. I pay by card so I'll have cash for the takeout. Were my sister a different sort of person, thirty euros would have covered both the Chinese food and the Pakistani corner store, but no, she's always had her nose in the air. Today she'll stoop to eating Chinese because she saw on some cop show that it's an ideal food for nights when you don't sleep. Maybe she'll let me make coffee, which she never drinks. Coffee is to her what pork is to Jews. She doesn't eat pork either, not because she's Jewish, but because her catechism is exceedingly strict about food. The one meat she tolerates is white meat, but only organic and in very small quantities. Drat, I've just realized I'll have to eat the beef noodle stir-fry by myself. Whatever, I like it. In fact, I love it. I love all red meat. I'm a huge fan of cadaverines and putrescines. Decomposing amino acids, a top-notch source of life! I'll have to convince her that the Chinese chicken is actually organic. No intensive poultry farming in the suburbs, no antibiotics or fast-growth hormones – this Chinese chicken is one hundred percent homemade. It was raised in the bathtub of an overcrowded migrant apartment and fed on leftover fried rice. It makes no difference whether she believes it. Tonight, my sister will eat anything. A blow to the self-esteem leaves a deep but non-lethal wound, a black hole that can suck up scraps of death and memory.

16

"You know I cannot marry you. We are lesbians!" I exclaim in English. Veronika smiles. "Of course you can! Since January 30 January!" Oh, putain. The legalization of gay marriage was a big win, don't get me wrong, but I'd been getting on just fine without it. Like coral snakes, not all marriages are poisonous – though it's best to keep your distance, just in case. For the sake of precision, a non-poisonous coral snake is called a false coral, which says it all.

I have something I need to say: I am not a sincere person. No, I'm someone who lies. I've been lying for as long as I can remember. All the time, every day, and almost without thinking – it's practically second nature to me. I lie so often I sometimes suspect I'm pathological. The truth is it has such a small effect on my day-to-day that I don't see why I should do anything about it. On that point, I've just arrived at the conclusion that I lie to make life easier for myself. Now that I think of it – God bless writing – I realize I tell three kinds of lies: accommodating lies, evasive lies, and weighty lies. The fact that I'm alive at all is thanks to them. Lies are the ancient logs over which my life glides; I just have to grab the ones in the back and put them in front again without stopping. Deep down, I'm a slave to myself. But the day will come when I can't take it anymore, and on that day the slave will die, not the other woman but the one everybody knows, the one who isn't me and yet seems openly to live my life. She is a heart in chains. Hearts are born in chains. It's a mistake to follow your heart while believing in your freedom, because freedom is the domain of lies. There, I said it. Lying is an act of resistance, a strategy of false appearances for the socially meek like me. Accommodating lies allow us to exist alongside the objectionable parts of reality, while evasive lies circumvent explanations and keep to a minimum all communication with unwelcome people or, under unwelcome circumstances, communication with people in general. And weighty lies, well, weighty lies prevent any harsh judgments from being passed on one's person. I am aware that these lies cleave to a brutal fear. But brutal fear can also be a driving force, and it has the astonishing ability to capsize the sturdiest relationships. Maybe this is why I refuse to establish any emotional ties. Christ, listen to me. Modern psychobabble is like methadone for imbeciles! I'll just give an example. Weighty lie: "Marry me!" Veronika is as stunning as ever. We've fucked all afternoon like animals on the verge of extinction. If I were male, I definitely would have gotten her pregnant. My entire body is a stick of hot, dense chewing gum tailored to her every cavity, searching for the point where the outside gives way to the naked and intimate inner pulp. I yearn for her essence, to meld with it. There is love so enormous it precludes the word love. Lips, hands and fingers, nose, tongue and feet, teeth, hair – and my clitoris, shockingly tripled in size, an insolent micropenis . . . my every extremity driven inside her, to the very edge of her, on the rack of unlimited desire. (I wonder now why there are such extremes of existential finitude to which death can't even aspire. Death requires solitude to exert power, but love and solitude are mutually exclusive relations. I'll have to rethink my own death, then, later on.) "You know I cannot marry you. We are lesbians!" Veronika smiles. Of course we can. We've been able to since last January. But even if we couldn't, "marry me" is the purest vow of permanence. A very fine glass shivers inside me and then splinters into painful shards. Veronika places between us a small, perfect box of chocolates with the Godiva ribbon and an embossed gold seal. I don't want to open it; I think of opening it. "Marry me, my love." Inside are my favorite chocolates and a beautiful, fat ring made of strange gold and encoded with drawings. I cry on the inside. "I can't," I say. She begins to cry too, without losing her composure, in silence. But it can't be. "There's another woman in my life," I lie. Every part of her was a cry for life. While my life was a cry for death.

17

"What do you mean, exactly, by 'with a woman?' What's it like to fuck a woman?" I ask. Of course that's what my sister means, but she gapes at me like a flounder. "I've just broken up with Ian!" she cries – or rather spits out, in the hope of hitting an emotional bullseye that I do not possess. I settle down next to her on the sofa. The white pleather squeaks like sneakers on a gym floor every time I sit, so I do my best to avoid it. I grab a piece of gum from the packet, pop it in my mouth, and start chewing. An otherworldly chill makes me drool like a poisoned dog. I've got to focus. I chew quickly to get past that critical moment when the artificial sweeteners assail the front line of the buccal cells. I try to get my bearings. I'll need that guest room for a few months, so I have to concentrate. "You're right, I'm sorry," I say. Thanks to this harmless, accommodating lie, my sister's usual self-pity is restored, and she slumps down at my side, the Ágatha Ruiz de la Prada flower tissue box cradled in her lap. She strokes it like she would a cat – tersely and with stiff fingers, fumblingly loving – then rests her head on my chest, ready for story time. I hope the Chinese food won't take long. My sister's hair looks clean but gives off an oily smell that reminds me of a churrería and makes me suuuuper uncomfortable. "Do you remember that movie we saw when we were little?" I begin. "*The Great Escape* – we watched it with Dad at least seven or eight times. It was about these American pilots in a German POW camp who dig this long, long tunnel that runs the length of the compound. But, on the night of the escape, when they reach the end of the tunnel, they realize they're six meters short of the forest. Their calculations had been off by six meters! They've got no choice but to risk their necks and make a run for it, in plain view of the guards. Do you remember?" "No," she says indifferently. "Whatever. What I'm trying to say is: Being with a woman is like sticking your head out of the tunnel and discovering that you've actually dug through those last few meters."

18

Getting a job after someone's put in a good word for you must be the closest thing to falling in love. You settle into a weightlessness that is for a while deeply pleasing, as though your life's been whisked down a tree-lined promenade that crests at a bridge over still water. As you gaze at green mallards and their single-parent families, you let go. It's so painless at the end of the day. And there's so much beauty, born again in your own face, permeating the friendly halves of other people. Your senses are honed. You rediscover the sun, whose light shines all around you and falls over exteriors like geometric shapes at rest. I don't see how this state of being can be normal. If it were, I might not be so shocked by everyone's eagerness to go on living day after day. But nothing can possibly be so long-lasting. The future awaits, a deer stopped on a country road. There's no doubt in my mind that an animal stopped on a road is suicidal. For those who can't seem to find *Amanita phalloides*, there's always Russian roulette on the highway. It's foolproof! I considered Russian roulette once, but then I pictured myself holding a gun and knew I would burst out laughing – new things always make me giggle. Maybe this is the source of my constant searching, of my rodent soul. And then there's the bit about having to take good aim to make sure you don't miss. I bet pulling a trigger requires some brawn in the index finger. It looks easy on TV – but then again, so do orgasms. And even I – and I happen to excel at them – recognize they require some basic knowledge, a certain degree of intelligence, because sex happens in the brain. The only vaginal orgasms I've ever had happened while I was asleep, all manner of women penetrating my vagina with deformed hands, like pig's trotters. Whenever I have these dreams, I wake up mid-orgasmic ecstasy. Curiously, I never dream of death. My subconscious seems only to want to travel and to fuck. I spend nights in hotel rooms, camping tents, caravans, cars, and stagecoaches. Never on planes. I have a lot of sex with strangers, and, funnily, these women and I are impressively in tune throughout. I can't complain. My brain's not a bad place to spend the night.

19

I'm ten or eleven years old and it's been an eye-opening day. In fact, it's been a whole month of eye-opening days. I've just learned that humans reproduce like animals. Like mammals! When the male's penis is hard and longer than usual, he sticks it in the female's vagina. Not only once but countless times, and very fast. Blinkingly quick. It doesn't count unless it happens that way. It sounds like the act itself isn't painful, but, suspiciously, it makes people scream. When he's done, the male spits semen through a tube in the penis, the same one he uses for peeing. He spits *inside* the female vagina. It's so gross – no, it's nasty! My girlfriends and I talk about it at school. We're so turned off we decide not to have children, but to adopt them from China instead. We are united by a revulsion that we extend to our mothers and fathers. Had they really done that? Some of us have brothers and sisters. Had Mom and Dad really done that *two* (sometimes even *three*) times? Later, the science teacher assigns us a project on tectonic plates. There are five kids in my group: two boys and three girls. We go to Laura's house. Laura is the most popular girl in our sixth-grade class. Actually, she's the most popular girl in the whole of sixth grade, groups A and B, the only blue-eyed blonde in a sea of brown-eyed brunettes. Besides, she plays the piano and has a parakeet that flies around the house whenever it feels like it. The thing that makes her most special, though, is the fact that her mom works. *Outside* the house. Sometimes when Laura comes home from school, she's alone until supper. Laura lets herself in with a key that hangs on a silver chain around her neck. We file in behind her, a little excited and a little sheepish, because we know no one's going to be watching us this afternoon. No grown-ups. This hardly ever happens, unless you're Laura. Laura acts as though she's older than us and says we can leave our backpacks in her bedroom, then shepherds us into the kitchen. Her mother has left us bollycaos and a bottle of Zumosol orange juice on the marble countertop. Laura suggests we eat our snacks on the living-room sofa with the TV on. We all grab the bollycaos, juice, cups, and some paper towels and set them on the glass coffee table in front of the TV. Laura asks if we'd like to watch one of her parents' videotapes. She's sure we'll like it. Nervous laughter. Bashful *yes*es. I think we should do our homework, but the prospect of watching a movie on a weekday is thrilling. This sort of thing never happens at home. It must be amazing to have movies in the house to watch whenever you like. Laura slides the tape into the VCR slit, which slurps it in. We all wait, wolfing down the chocolaty bollycaos with our eyes glued to the screen. The first images appear. I haven't seen this movie before. I have an excellent memory for movies, and I can't remember ever watching one that opens with a party in a swimming pool. Laura grabs the clicker and fast-forwards the tape at full speed. "What're you doing?" asks Ivan. I'm outraged too. You can't jump ahead like that. "Hang on, I'm just skipping the boring bits." She pauses the tape abruptly and presses play. A silent tension rises immediately from each of us and we band together in an extraordinary conspiracy. Onscreen, a naked woman shamelessly flashes her shaven genitals. Her hair is bleached and held back with a

headband across her forehead. She wears a lot of makeup –
her eyes are painted green, her cheeks pink, and her lips
fuchsia. She has on huge gold hoop earrings. Her skin is dark
like it's the end of summer and she's spent every day lying
naked by that pool. She has enormous breasts and nipples
the size of a roll of Scotch tape. Her breasts sway from side
to side and are just how I want mine to be when I grow up.
The woman lies on a pool chair. Rather, the woman lies on
a man who is lying on a pool chair, spread-eagled with knees
bent. Though the man's face is hidden, the fact that he's
furry all over and has a penis means he is obviously a man.
His penis is massive. Gigantic! It's much larger than a dog's,
which is how I imagined men's penises to look, though not
as long. I'm breathless. The man keeps on penetrating the
woman, back and forth, back and forth. The entire screen is
a close-up of that pinkish, slimy penis slipping in and out of
the woman's vagina. The woman pulls strange faces and
moans with her mouth wide open. Sergi laughs; the rest of
us are dead quiet. Laura glances at us and the TV in turn.
I know we're doing something we aren't supposed to, but
I can't and don't want to stop watching. It's horrifying – but
also phenomenal! Then, a third person comes on scene. Small
and beefy, he approaches the woman from the side. The man
is touching his penis! Holding it and rubbing it with his whole
hand like it's itchy, but only a little. He's doing it calm as can
be. With every rub his hand grows smaller and his penis
larger. When he reaches the woman, he does something that
stuns every single one of us. Well, except for Laura, who
smiles smugly, like it's the most natural thing in the world.
He puts his penis inside the woman's mouth. "Gross!" Anna
yells. I think I might retch, but instead my mouth goes dry.
Inside it, the morsel of bollycao turns hard and coarse, like
a clod of earth. "Do you want me to stop the tape?" Laura

asks. "No!" we answer in unison. The woman looks like she wants to eat the man's penis but never actually does. She just licks and swallows it with her lips, a fuchsia ring that circles his dick and adapts to its shape. It's astonishing. Veins like on an athlete's arm – green subcutaneous snakes – criss-cross the penis from end to end. It's wider at the base, like Obelix's menhir. Now and then, the man presses the tip of his penis with his fingers and out come droplets like liquid detergent for washing sweaters, thick and translucent, which he smears on the woman's lips with the tip of his cock before sticking it in her mouth again. It's not semen. We know semen is white because the eighth graders told us about it. What is it, then? None of what we're seeing has been explained in class. When it looks like the man's had enough, he gets between the woman's legs, placing his knees in the little space left on the pool chair, and penetrates her at the same time as the other guy. Both of them at the *same time*. I can't believe my eyes. That's got to be painful. In fact, the woman won't stop moaning or screaming, though she doesn't seem to actually object or do anything to get away. We think we've seen it all, and that's when it happens. The man under-neath her takes his penis out of her vagina and puts it in another hole, in front. "What's he doing?" Irene asks. "Come on! There's no way this is real," I blurt out. Women don't have two vaginas! Thank God the whole thing is fake. It has to be. "It's her asshole – can't you see?" said Sergi, disbeliev-ing. That's the last thing I remember from that afternoon. I assume at some point Laura stopped the video and we started on our science project. What I do remember is getting home and going to the bathroom to pee, wiping myself with a square of toilet paper, and discovering a clear, sticky sub-stance. I didn't make the connection with the movie – the first thought I had was that I must be sick, but I didn't want to explain anything to Mom. That night, I masturbated. Just like I'd done every night for the past couple of years. I masturbated in bed morning and night, systematically. I masturbated at other times, too – when I remembered, in our bathroom, or in the school restroom. That night, I didn't just rub my clitoris over my panties, like I usually did, but touched myself inside too. The sticky substance was still there, like alien drool. I was a little alarmed because the goo seemed to trap my fingers and suction them inward. Oddly, I didn't feel the slightest hint of pain. Maybe I wasn't sick. Out of curiosity, I took two damp fingers to my mouth. They were viscous, as if coated in a semi-liquid pastry glaze. And sweet, too! New, and exceptionally sweet, unlike any sugary food I'd ever eaten. Although the smell reminded me a little of fruit yogurt. I licked my fingers clean, then did it again: dunked my fingers inside and licked them. It dawned on me that this was the closest I would come to eating myself. This thought led naturally to another, like when you look up a word in the dictionary whose definition includes another word you don't know and have to look up. I wondered if it was the same for my friends, Marta and Anna. And I wondered especially about Laura, who wasn't really a friend, even though I would've liked her to be my best friend. Then I wondered what it would feel like to dunk my fingers into Laura's fig, what she would taste like. Sweet and fruity like me? Or sweet and sour like those heart-shaped candies she was always eating during recess? One day, Laura gave Marta and me one to share and it was the most amazing thing I'd ever tasted. The candy was soft but chewy and coated in tart, lemony sugar that melted on the tongue and left a much tangier aftertaste than any ordinary sugar. These thoughts made my body produce more of that viscous substance. It soaked my fingers and spilled from the opening, all the way up and over my clitoris. I'd known for some weeks that the thing I fondled through my panties when masturbating was called a clitoris, but now that I was touching it directly with fingers smeared in juice, the pleasure I felt was a thousand times more intense. Or ten thousand times! I climaxed almost instantly, without having to chase it. The thought of Laura's syrupy fig immediately made me come. I licked my fingers, savored them, and started over. Three or four times in a row. Until my clitoris, practically numb, began to tingle almost painfully. I stopped and fell asleep thinking of Laura. I kissed the line between my index finger and thumb. I pictured them as her lips, slipped my tongue between them, and wondered whether one day, maybe when we were older, Laura would let me do the same to her fig. It was a fantastic discovery and I felt sorry for the woman in the movie with the headband and the huge hoop earrings who had to settle for the juices of that small, beefy man, served up in a pipette.

20

It started as a small dot, like a black speck of sand that sticks to the skin and is impossible to get off. It turned up smack in the middle of my stomach, four fingers above my belly button. I found it strange – it was so centered – and I felt proud to have produced something so unique right on my line of symmetry. Three weeks later, it had grown a little. It was round and black like an eclipse, and had a bright halo, as though it had cast its harsh darkness on the surrounding skin, intensifying its whiteness. I was fond of it. I found it beautiful. A remarkable mole less than two millimeters across, which is how it stayed for about a year or two. Then, one day, all of a sudden, it began to grow again, fast, like a plant that shoots up after being spiked with fertilizer. "It's those cheap moisturizers you use," my sister chided. Mom also weighed in. "It's the sun. Did you know that the sun's cancerous rays can pierce through up to four layers of clothing? Even in winter?" Cancerous rays? "Honest, Mom, I don't think I could wear four layers in the summer." "You know what I mean. Because the sun feels weaker in the winter, we underestimate how cancerous it is, but people should really be applying high-factor sunscreen all year long. And all over their bodies!" Life really is full of surprises. "On the soles of their feet, too?" I said for a laugh. "Of course! Did you know foot melanoma is the skin cancer with the worst survival rates?" Quite the oncologist, my mother. "Jesus, Mom. Give it a rest, will you?" Who knew, maybe luck was on my side. A death by melanoma was a death worth considering. A word so close to "melomaniac" and "megalomaniac" couldn't be that bad, a slight etymological violation. "You should make an appointment to see the dermatologist. At a private practice. It'll have spread to your internal organs by the time you're seen to at a public clinic." A sensible idea. I mulled it over for a few days, then made an appointment with a public health physician.

21

"We've decided you should be our witness." "Witness to what?" "Our wedding, of course!" I can't believe my ears. My sister is what people call radiant. But what exactly radiates? She gazes at me with an immaculate smile. The skin on her cheeks reminds me of the worn knee of a porcelain Baby Jesus. As a kid, I'd been an altar girl at Midnight Mass. One of my tasks was to hold fake Baby Jesus before a line of parishioners who'd come to kiss him on the knee. Sometimes there were up to two thousand people and they'd bend over him one by one. Between kisses, I wiped Baby Jesus's knee with a small altar cloth. I took it very seriously, rubbing and rubbing until finally the priest hissed in my ear: the cloth's just symbolic, you're not trying to erase a chalkboard! Symbolic, my ass. Some lipsticks really do have a lasting touch, and Catholicism couldn't give a damn. Take the part where everyone drinks the blood of Christ from the same cup. Holy germ-sharing! I was only an altar girl for a year before I was let go, which was unprecedented and, to be honest, quite the relief. I've always thought of unprecedented dismissals as strokes of genius from higher powers. I picture Lachesis sidestepping her scissor-handed sister. I should give serious thought to a tête-à-tête with Lachesis; her older sister deserves a lot of respect. "I'm getting married!" my own sister announces. "Who's the lucky guy?" "I won't let you ruin my day with your stupid jokes. Here." She hands me a piece of paper with the date, location, and time, then explains that I will serve as their witness at City Hall a few days before the wedding. I will, in other words, be their shadow witness. They'll have proper witnesses on the wedding day. At least she's a considerate bitch, my sister. "What have you done to your face?" I ask. "Teeth whitening and two chemical peels. It really shows, doesn't it?" She bares her teeth and smiles like a horse. The end result is outstanding, pediatric white up to the canines. "Shame about the mercury fillings," I say. She's only got one in a bottom molar, and it flashes when she smiles the way she's smiling now. "Well, it's not like I'm going to walk into church with my mouth hanging open, am I?" she says. "Church? You're getting married in a church?" Though I wouldn't put it past my sister to tie the knot in a temple, I'd have thought a Catholic church would be her last choice. I could sooner picture her wed at a biosphere reserve, a ziggurat, a Shinto shrine, on a beach in Formentera, a Zen cave, in a Buddhist temple, a pyramid, or at Stonehenge. Even a synagogue, at a push. But a church? "Of course. We want our wedding to be romantic, not just some bureaucratic appointment in a seedy corner of City Hall, like we've gone to register the dog or request a real estate deed." Registering a dog? Conversations with my sister are a never-ending source of inspiration. I think of Paul Klee's *A Tiny Tale of a Tiny Dwarf*. He probably had a sister like mine. A shame I never did get that fine arts degree. I've got a sister as untapped as a Christmas hamper at my mother's house.

22

She was French. Marseillaise, actually, like the national anthem. The nerve center of her beauty resided in her being French. I was in love with her nationality, a second face with perfect features cast over the first like a semitransparent film, but with the charm of the great classics. Her name was Roxanne and she was shorter than me, slimmer than me, more intelligent and nobler than me. She was more educated, too: a PhD in literature with diplomas in English, German, and Italian. On top of all of that, she was magnificent on the piano. She had one at home in a large room that I pompously referred to as the piano room and where she played long pieces from memory. She was, as Mom would put it, from a good family, and this being-from-a-good-family showed on her like a coat of varnish. In fact, it showed in every single gesture, no matter how insignificant. For example, she had a particular way of moving her chin when opening the door, lifting it very slightly to one side while casting her eyes down, and I always felt like she took for granted that someone would step aside for her. It's hard to explain – but it was obvious when I saw it. She was a climber and though at the time I couldn't imagine my life without her, the moment I saw her naked body, I decided all my future lovers should have loved climbing in their past. Her muscles were perfect, thrumming and covered in supple, impeccable skin. Her every position in bed was an anatomical study in red chalk – improbably precise and as exciting as a first visit to Casa Buonarroti. I remember her stomach – quiet and commanding like a tortoise shell – and the tensed arch of her arms, her ass, her thighs and her calves – compact like thinking skulls – all centered on me and my pleasure alone, on reaching the summit of my pleasure. Never before nor since have I spent so many nights screwing. By that I mean whole nights, five or six or seven hours of relentless fucking, mostly with her on top. "Talk to me in French," I would ask. And she'd say some things I understood and others I didn't have to understand. It was enough just to listen to her, to let her words penetrate my body, softening it in strange and unpredictable ways. Her voice shook me violently, consumed me, a wisp of hair singed by a cigarette ember. My body shrank and coiled at once, assaulted by her accent like a doughy maggot being pricked by a pin. As I write this, I relive it, and millions of my cells pass along buckets of glowing water to put out goodness knows what fire. Fast and blind. My heart flares up, damaging the pleural membrane, which is so unaccustomed to playing along. Roxanne. When I met her, she'd just bought a professional camera. I envied the camera for spending all day in her hands, white with slender knuckles and polished tips. Before playing the piano, she used to splay her fingers over the keys, and it was as if they were simply resting for a moment, both contained and laid out, like a row of matching surgical tools before a very delicate intervention. Then she would subtly flex them and move them according to instructions from a series of neck muscles triggered milliseconds before her fingers. I listened as the sound of the piano strings penetrated me like her words, shaking me and giving rise to inexplicable surges and a sort of self-indulgent jealousy. I followed the unintelligible movement of her fingers as they drove the composition toward the moment when it would finally die out. She adored Satie. "It's easy," she said. And over and over she played "Je te veux," the first "Gymnopédie," and the second "Nocturne." "They're so long," I'd grumble. And she would laugh and retort, "They're only three minutes," then play them again. And I renewed myself in that image, of my French piano-playing lover. But every second I died. And it was a very dignified, respectable way to go.

23

"So, what's it like with a woman? In bed, I mean." It's half past twelve and it's taken my sister two whole servings of almond chicken and fried rice to let her hair down. Or maybe it was the Coke. She hasn't had any in more than three years. Slow-acting poison, she calls it. But tonight is special. Not everybody has a lesbian sister to comfort them after a breakup. Tonight's heart-to-heart will be a real treat – irresistibly modern, maybe even obscene. My sister can't help picturing herself as the lead in a popular TV series. Playing the sister of the lesbian is quite the role; it offers a seal of respectability. "Do you want Nestea?" I ask her before dinner. She throws me a thunderous look, as if she'd just decided to go into business with the mafia. "Screw it, I'll have the Coke!" she says, thrilled. Screw it! "Careful it doesn't go to your head. You're not used to such strong beverages." My sister doesn't know her way around a can, so I transfer the Coke into a tall glass that she takes from my hands with a wanton gleam in her eye. The poor thing feels funny, she's used to getting her beauty sleep. But great things are afoot! "What's it like" – enticing inquiry – "to fuck a woman?" I swear this is the first time she's ever uttered the word "fuck," plumb-drunk on Coca-Cola. "So that's what you wanted to know?" I ask with a dash of cruelty. I flat-out refuse to suffer fools, even when they try to make an effort. "You know that's not true!" she cries. I concentrate on the guest room and nothing but the guest room, crucial as fingernails. "Shall I tell you another story?" She nods with a headful of eyes and the aspartame-laced smiles of a pampered girl who will never, never-ever indulge in another can of Coke. "All right," I consent. The tactic works. "Have you ever heard of action painting?" Now she shakes her head. "Jackson Pollock?" I insist. "No." "Okay." I walk into my room and bring out a book of Pollock paintings. It's tremendous; images like these make me reevaluate my love affair with death. "This is art? A child could have made these!" my sister blurts. "But a child didn't." The woman must be dumb. Thick as two planks. This guest room is costing me a tidy sum, but what else can I do? Where else can I go? The glutamate in the sweet-and-sour prawns is affecting my ability to think, but I have another go. I'm sure that with some effort I can pluck a plastic flower from the dunghill, a plastic flower that will satisfy the dregs of curiosity of the poor aborted lesbian lurking in my sister's brain. "This is an action painting," I begin. "Action painting is the product of impatience." She pulls a face like a cricket. "Around the mid-twentieth century, there was a period when artists were no longer being challenged. For centuries, they'd struggled with a series of problems: motif, depth, form, color, realism, fidelity, light . . . everything! In other words, they'd run out of lines of inquiry. And then Pollock rocked up with his huge, unplanned canvases stretched out on the floor, and wham!" "Wham?" "Look at this." I show her *Number 3*, flip pages, *Number 5*, flip pages, *Number 34*, a superb piece with that horrific red-thinking head and its two yellow hemispheres. "Look," I tell her. "Clear, simple manipulation of raw material! Pure experimentation! Pollock splattered canvases driven by the spontaneity of the moment. A work of art isn't only the end result – it's art in time, art in real time, in action, as simple and impulsive as a drawing by a child. But there's a sophisticated concern below the surface, an interest in process – life's immensity concentrated in that process. Do you get what I'm saying?" "Sort of." "All right. So now you sort of know what it's like to fuck a woman."

24

Seven months had passed. Enough for it to have metastasized? I had no idea. The mole's growth had slowed. The bottom edge of its beautiful contour had blotted. Once a deep black, it was now a faded brown, consummated in a series of tiny specks that no longer formed part of the raised cluster but existed as solitary, pigmented entities hovering a few millimeters below what could still be considered the mole. To be safe, I canceled my appointment with the dermatologist and started the process from scratch. Ahead of me lay ten more months of waiting, ten months for the altered cells to migrate – not downward, but deep inside.

25

I always suspected that Roxanne was more suicidal than I was. That she would die first, I had no doubt, but most of all, that her desire for death had hardened within her into a formative whole. I was also convinced that she would die a more elegant death. Someone inside her was burnishing every single thing she did, every measured word she said – but who? Catalan phrases strutted out of her throat wrapped in French-accented mink, but with a lowly, port-like fragrance that I attributed to her Marseilles roots and which drove me wild. In her mouth, Catalan sounded the way it should sound as a perfect language. Any word that I said immediately afterward was a faded daisy in comparison, a silly little flower. I've never spoken as sparingly as I did with her, and I've never enjoyed the lead-in to a conversation quite as much. Whenever she opened her lips with a click of the tongue that recalled a book whose pages lay open under a strong wind, my heart would turn so slick it became an organ out of control. Every beat, every deliberate whiplash of life was trapped inside it. And it wasn't just my chest, either. Every part of me flared up under the influence of her words. "*Què vols sopar?*" she'd ask. And she would say it just like that, in italics, because she had the ability to apply font to speech. She did it every time, and without realizing. It made me dizzy. "*Encara queda Camembert del que vaig portar ahir?*" And I was reduced to aftershocks of pleasure, at whose epicenter was the word "Camembert." I tried my best to say something, stressing the paroxytones in an effort to appear interesting. "Of course. I had salmon for lunch so we could have the Camembert for dinner." Lies. Big. Fat. Lies. I'd had sausage and beans, except I couldn't be with Roxanne and also be someone who ate sausage and beans. Absolutely not. I would have sausage for lunch, air out the apartment, take the trash down to the dumpster, and claim I had salmon. Because even though salmon isn't Camembert, it belongs to the same part of the pyramid as the foods I used to save for days when I wanted to treat myself, as Mom likes to put it, before I met Roxanne. This never made sense to Roxanne, whose whole life was a treat. Roxanne often had croissants for breakfast – flakey on the outside, insides soft, buttery, and still warm. She bought them from a bakery four blocks from her house, where they were held for her. She drank coffee like I did, but not just any old coffee. She had her coffee delivered from a shop where it was ground sur place seconds before being packaged. She didn't have ordinary ham; she had smoked ham. When we ate at her place, she would cook a peculiar type of pasta that looked like a ruddy, serrated snail shell, sautéed with hot spices and served with sprout salad. She loved funky cheeses. She filled my fridge with Comté, Brie, Époisses de Bourgogne, Gaperon, and Roquefort, none of which were labeled the way they usually were in supermarkets, if they stocked them in the first place. She got a different brand every time, each more authentic than the last, and imported. The same could be said of everything about her – her clothes, her hobbies, the building she lived in, her hair. She wore a single piece of jewelry: a striated ring the width of one finger on the middle finger of her right hand. She almost always dressed in dark clothes. She had pale skin and liked to wear baggy sweaters with long sleeves that fell halfway down her hand. I used to dream about those sweaters. I would dream of her white, silver-ringed hand as it emerged from a deep-blue sleeve, cold and slow like a sea mollusk. My eyes would fixate on her hand as it stirred pasta in the wok with the chopsticks she usually used to cook. I was captivated by that finger, her ring finger. It was perhaps her only concession to traditional constructs of femininity. Even though everything about her screamed femininity: head blonde and shorn like a solid and recently shaven cunt, cracked-ice eyes, breasts long and continuous like tongues resting over a flight of ribs, crimped nipples, legs and feet soft and monochrome like the drawings in the classical Kama Sutra. Her flesh was taut, smooth, and moderately full, her mouth wild like a natural cleft in a chunk of mineral rock, and her tongue . . . her tongue was a sovereign being that lived alongside her, a slave to my pleasure. It talked to me and fucked me and carried on talking while Roxanne fucked me instead, a partially domesticated animal, dogged and feral when entering my cunt. She hadn't wanted to at first. "I love it when you eat me out," she said on our first night together, "though I don't usually do it myself." "You'd better start." Pleasure is a lower value, but Scheler had a knack for changing sides and change can be an excellent source of knowledge. She did it. It became her favorite part, in fact. She could keep at it all evening, like a lioness fixated on a wound. A slow, rhythmical licking. And I struck back. Our cunts were our favorite set of fine china. We plated them with fruit salad – segments of mandarin and sweet orange, which we peeled and sliced into pieces. We held fruit in our lips and between our teeth, dipped the pieces inside ourselves and fed them to one another. Now and then we doused each other in chocolate syrup or raspberry sauce, and if we spotted a seed, we would tuck it into the folds of our lips or lick it into the hole. Wiping myself after peeing the next day, I might come across a seed and smile. Innocent little seed, in a pee stain, on a piece of toilet paper. A childlike gemstone of immeasurable worth.

26

"It's a girl! Her name is Arlet and you're going to be her godmother." My sister, seconds after my mother passes her the phone. Out of the question. "Aren't godparents meant to look after the kid if the parents die?" I ask. No newborn deserves a suicidal godmother. They've only just been tossed into the world; their asses are still see-through and their shit slimy like crude oil, their whole selves an interrogation, an open, circling question mark punctuated by a dot. No way, I don't give a damn if the kid's my sister's. "No, dumbass, the godmother's the one who bakes La Mona de Pascua. And it's a girl. Also, we're not planning on dying. And if we did end up in a fatal accident, do you think we'd leave you the kids? You? They need the stability of a marriage." Fatal accident, a stunning pair of words. Porphyry believed that an accident was something which became present, then absent without destroying its subject. A fatal accident could therefore be contradictory. I picture my sister in a hospital bed with chrome side rails, her hair filthy from giving birth, her skin greasy, dressed in a white gown with pink polka dots over a stomach landsliding underneath, the baby breastfeeding, amniotic residue crammed in the folds of her neck and wrists, a little rancid, like a steak tray in the night trash, untouchable, an abhorrent stump in place of the belly button, tender and clamped with one of those plastic clips used to seal cereal bags. Untouchable but loved, of course. Loved from the very first moment, with her pierced little ears and her name. Names are our first possession and they're as painful, if not more, than a piercing. "What if I meet the woman of my dreams and get married?" I ask. "Even if you get married, children need the stability of two parents. A mother and a father. I don't want you to take this the wrong way, but . . . do you see what I'm saying?" The miserable cow. It's easier than she thinks to see what she's saying. But trying to understand her is about as attractive as the thought of breeding worms in an ulcer. As far as my sister is concerned, the only stability a lesbian can offer is baking La Mona de Pascua cake for Easter.

27

I am twelve years old. I've grown up, and everything to do with sex – or at least, the sex other people have – is a bit less taboo. People don't realize this, but apparently sex works the same as coffee or certain kinds of food: When you're little, your palate isn't fully developed. The adults laugh and tell you that once you've grown up, you'll learn to appreciate caviar, curry, or goulash, that it comes with time, it really does. I figured the same had to apply to having sex with boys because both the sex I had on my own and the sex I had in my head – featuring my girlfriends, girls in the older kids' class, the occasional teacher or actress, and the women depicted in the art books we had at home – was brilliant, without comparison, perfect, and delicious. I loved it! And the fact that I liked it so much could mean only one thing: that it was kid-friendly sex, like having macaroni and lollipops for lunch. Or, at a stretch, that it was teenage-friendly sex: Pop Rocks and Kit Kats. I knew for sure that I would have to mature before I acquired a taste for sex with boys. The man-on-woman sex scenes I saw on TV didn't turn me off. In fact, I found them as arousing, maybe even more so, than the porn we had watched at Laura's house. But what about them, exactly, aroused me? At twelve years old, I'd been privy to very few erotic scenes. Maybe twenty, tops. Sometimes they cropped up without warning during a Saturday night movie, and I would sit, still and painfully quiet, sheltered by the very tall upholstered backrest of my armchair with the tiny dragonflies on it, more aware than ever of my parents on the sofa behind my sister and me, watching what we were watching. Didn't they realize their ten- and twelve-year-old daughters were in the room with them? They acted like it was nothing, while a hard, prickly silence filled the dining room. I held my breath so that it filled me from head to toe – because in a way their silence excluded me, and this made it painful. At the same time, I committed the movie scene to memory – not just the characters kissing and touching one another, but also the context. I found it arousing to project myself into that same situation, beside the same woman; I nearly always played the role of the man. Take *Dangerous Liaisons*. For years I recreated that iconic movie, night in and night out. I was the Vicomte de Valmont, stealing into the chambers of the delectable Cécile de Volanges to convince her of the inevitable desecration of her innocence, satiating my desire with her body, virginal and inexperienced but, above all, receptive to the pleasure I gave her. I reconstructed this scene a thousand and one times in the darkness of my bedroom, reenacting it and tacking on variations. The crisp white bedsheets, the sheer and delicate fabric of the nightgowns, the garnet velvet of the canopy, Uma Thurman's long, blonde mane and her parted lips, which I forced open with my fine and experienced tongue, or the black, wavy hair of my English teacher and her breasts like giant castanets shaken by her gasps, large and soft beneath a yellow blouse like the one she had worn that morning in class – except longer, tumbling down to her ankles – and which I pushed up with one hand, forcing it between her thighs. I did the same to Michelle Pfeiffer as Madame de Tourvel and to Vanessa – beautiful, tentative Vanessa, who had started at our school halfway through the year and sat next to me in class. And so on, with many more women and many more movies.

28

I'm not a sex addict, though I do spend a lot of the day thinking about sex. I picture sexual encounters and imagine what
it would be like to have sex with attractive women I pass on
the street. I masturbate almost every night and am never
without a lover for longer than two or three months. Sex
distances me from death, though it doesn't bring me closer to
life. What, then? For what? Having thought it over for a few
minutes, I arrive at the conclusion that sex keeps me present
and safe in a space both uncertain and comforting. Why do
I feel the need to be there? I don't know. It's not that I want
to die, but that I have to. It's my truth. Life belongs to others,
it always has. I am here and I see it passing, life passes by
other lives; life is a mirage that is real and unfathomable, and
it flows through the lives of others, sating them with water,
bloating them into double chins. The fact that my turn had
come was an accident. Not an accident à la Porphyry – not
this time – but logical in a neoscholastic sense. My life is an
accident, predicable and transgressive. It gives no ontolog-
ical meaning to my existence, but rather occupies it like a
sentinel, where it grows strong and renders me absolute.
Self-justified, life destroys me. I think a lot about sex, but
I also think about heights, train tracks, Gillette razors, Swiss
Army knives, and kitchen knives; about barbiturates, pools,
and bathtubs; about acid, psychopaths, armed robbers, flags,

and red traffic lights. I think about highways, wrong ways, high bridges, falling flowerpots, rabid dogs, and rattlesnakes. I think a lot about terrorist attacks and medical errors, about oxygen-filled syringes, unforeseen landslides, controlled avalanches, chasms, and hidden wells. I think about eggs long past their expiration date, alcohol poisoning, and deer traps; about rats under the cover of night and worn-out steps; about old mines, stray bullets, and brain MRIs; about cramps at high sea and sharks that have lost their way. I think about all of these things while also having to put up with my enemy, my trained kamikaze, as impatient and vexing as leaven.

29

My subconscious has excellent survival instincts, which is odd, considering my dreams often drop me into situations of extreme peril. In dreams, death takes the shape of long, flat animals like snakes, crocodiles, and scorpions, though lately I've found myself repeatedly faced with serial killers, chainsaw-wielding lunatics, nooses, firearms of every caliber, and knife sets in rolls like the ones on *Top Chef*. I also visit places in the throes of natural disasters, floods and volcanic eruptions in particular. I'm there almost every night. When I dream, a second consciousness is switched on and works at full throttle, and I am filled with the conviction that my being there is not real at all but that I am actually asleep and can behave in ways that are unusual, unexpected. At least, this is what my first consciousness wants; I know because this is what it thinks. My physical presence in dreams is simple and improbably crisp, like a medieval illustration in an incunable at the British Library with primary colors pure as can be; the body invisible and solemn, face rigid, practically Egyptian, yet open thanks to eyes wider than they have ever been and hands whose two fingers – the ones usually used to nudge the ovum deep inside the cunt – are raised in warning, like in images of grown-up angels, and feet – feet bare and hovering centimeters above the head of an enormous snake. I think, Reach your foot down! Tread on the Crotalus!

Put your hand in the basket like a Cleopatra freshly arrived in the nineteenth century, in her white-and-green rental cottage in Chantilly. But I refuse to listen; I am a rebellious daughter – against everyone, even myself – and hateful to the point of causing miscarriage. Stop! I tell myself. Face up to the man with panties on his head! Kick him in the balls while flashing him your jugular and let him sink his saw into you like butter! Or sit on this rock and let the lava burn your ass to a crisp. Do it! Get a taste of death – then you'll know. You'll know what the hell is keeping you from taking the next step. Imminence is just the carrot dangled by the future to keep us present. I fall for it all the time. And I chase after it, too, because freedom in death is an outstanding slogan and I'm nuts about slogans. I'm savvy, so savvy that I can't wait, even though a split second is always tempting. The days pass, and my life as it is portrayed puckers like a caterpillar, then advances – not as real as the lives of others but submerged like the crew on a U-boat, ever on the lookout and ever alert. And yet it behaves like all the others, and, though I can hardly believe it, I'm the one living it, feeding it. My instinct for self-preservation is so pronounced I should have been a scientist. And caught a hemorrhagic fever while I was at it.

30

She was a woman. By that, I mean a female rather than a male dermatologist. She wasn't attractive and yet the morning sun poured through the tall windows behind her with such force it seemed almost to penetrate her, magnifying her humanity and dressing her in a beauty that she certainly lacked outside the office. She'd just set beside her computer a small plastic cup rimmed with residues of coffee foam, and it occurred to me that her tongue must also be the intoxicated yellow that comes from drinking coffee. I was her first patient of the day. I'd arrived a little before eight and sat alone in the waiting room, rereading Kierkegaard and collecting myself. The doctor saw me right away. She was younger than me. Her white coat looked new and hung loose on her body. Next to the sink sat a small plant with a couple of buds about to bloom. That same morning, probably. She smiled at me and everything – her youth, her baggy coat, the plant, her smile – made me feel guilty. Did I really have to go and ruin this doctor's day? She seemed nice. What if this was her first case of melanoma diagnosed at a first consultation and during a first examination in a woman as young as I was? My mole was now more a meteor than a mole, a dark comet with a powerful trail of particles glowing behind it. Its suckerfish had multiplied in such a way that the entire mole seemed to have shifted, creeping a few centimeters up my stomach.

According to my mother's calculations, no less than a couple of colonies of malignant cells should have already taken root in some shimmering organ inside me. I wasn't concerned about the fact that I had no symptoms. I was sure they'd show before long, just as soon as I had a confirmed diagnosis. I prayed for it to be too late to get treatment; I preferred a sudden growth and a predictable end. "So, what can I help you with?" she asked, looking me square in the eyes. Hers were brown and they sparkled, as though her skull was a pumpkin and inside the flame of a candle was flickering. How could I get her to understand that I was beyond help? Without hurting her? Without snuffing out that lovely, animate, impermanent flame? In this woman? In vocation incarnate? In her white coat and *Sistine Madonna*-esque halo that the sharp light had drawn around her, filtered through the blinds? Did I really have to go and do that to her? On a morning bright enough to make buds bloom? Not me – I wasn't going to be the one to make her cry. "My doctor told me I should have some moles checked out," I said innocently. "Let's take a look then," she suggested. I followed the direction of her hand to the exam table. "Where should we start?" she asked excitedly, just as if we were at our wedding menu tasting. She wasn't attractive, and now that she'd stepped outside the light her whole body had dimmed a little. But she had very nice, comforting hands. "It's these ones," I said, unwrapping the green scarf with orange duck beaks from around my neck and sliding the collar of my shirt down a little. It's worth pointing out that I have an unconventional chest – inherited from my mother – with eight ruddy moles, shapeless and of varying size. These moles are not dainty moles. Three are clustered together in a primitive constellation like a pointy triangle at the base of my neck, a little off to the left. The other five look like someone shook them in a dice cup and scattered them on my chest. They're not a pretty sight, but I've had them since I was ten years old and I know for sure that they're harmless. Mom had had them looked at – at a private clinic, of course – and the doctor in question had assured us that my moles and I would live peaceably until the end of my days. The dermatologist lifted her hands to my collarbone. Both hands. A couple of fingers alighted, smooth as a seaplane. I pictured her in bed, touching me in that gentle and focused way, determined and skillful. Her fingers circled my moles like inquisitive creatures around an intruder of unknown species. They tugged my skin flat, then released it, and carefully fondled the moles' granular surface . . . wait a second. Was she actually fondling my moles? Without gloves? She was – she was touching them! I went into a state of shock. Not even I touched my moles with such intent. They were pretty unappealing. Did she not realize this? My sister had bullied me about them for most of my childhood, claiming that nobody would ever want me, that they'd turn huge and hairy like a cow's, that I'd have to wear a turtleneck to get anyone to fall in love with me and they'd still run away the moment they discovered my secret, leaving me all alone. For the rest of my life. "You've got no choice but to become a nun," she'd asserted somberly. I think she might have actually believed it. Unsung childhood trauma. Her words ate away at my liver until one day, she got moles too, on the inside of her arm, redder and bulgier than mine. For a few months, I had faith in the power of the mind – I'd infected her with them! I don't think I've ever been happier than the day her moles grew to the same size as mine, then kept growing until they were nearly twice as big. Next to them, my moles were shy little girls. Hers, on the other hand, reared up on pinker skin, like strange, cerise sandcastles in ruins. One summer, they started to peel. We were sitting on towels at the edge of the pool playing cards when I screamed, "Look!" then pointed at the largest mole, covered in a crust that looked like powdered sugar. She ran over to Mom, who comforted her and said they'd go see the doctor again. The doctor corroborated his previous diagnosis: totally harmless. Still, as a teenager, my sister had her moles removed. For psychological reasons, apparently. For similar reasons, I opted to keep mine. And there I was, ready to weaponize them. The dermatologist brought her lighted magnifying glass to my chest and lingered there a while, her face centimeters from my breasts, my head thrown back to keep out of her way. I could feel her breathing, I could feel her drawing oxygen from my pores and exhaling it as carbon dioxide, hot and heavy with viruses endemic to her bronchial tree. It occurred to me that inspections like this could be as infectious as an erotic encounter. "You don't have to worry about these moles," she said. She'd drawn away and sat before me on a swivel stool, legs wide, ready to get to the bottom of things. "How about we give you a general look-see while you're here?" A general look-see? That was not a medical term. The woman was so sweet, she didn't deserve to find out about my cancerous cells. "Go on, take your shirt off so I can check your back." It would have looked suspicious to refuse. I considered rolling up my shirt, bending over myself, and cradling my secret like a newborn while the doctor played with her magnifying glass, then getting shyly dressed and taking off before it was too late. I mean, too late for her and for her innocence, which was probably still intact. I did as she asked, and she ruled out the moles on my back. "There are a lot of them, but they're all perfectly normal," she assured me. Perfectly normal. If the moles on my back could become permanent to such an unnatural degree without questioning themselves, why couldn't I? "Let's check your belly." Belly, what belly? I turned to her. It was clear I was going to have to say something about my melanoma before she pegged me for an idiot. My mother and my sister were the only women I could bear to think of me as an idiot. "I've had this special mole for a while but it's never bothered me." Special? Eight in the morning, a perfect moment for dumb observations. I couldn't get out of it in the end. I felt bad for her. She would just have to diagnose me and refer me on to someone else. I focused my attention on the plant. Did she water it herself, or did the janitors? It looked like an African violet – stiff, meaty leaves, a coat of almost pubescent fuzz, and buds fair and tough like cherry pits. "This?" she asked, fondling the skin around the mole and pulling it up to the magnifying glass. Yes, I thought as I tried to make the flowers bloom from a distance. "Oh, this is nothing. Still, you should have them looked at – like the rest of them – at least once every couple of years." I let my head fall forward, stared at my stomach, and pointed at the shooting-star mole, thick with black, clearly cancerous suckerfish. "This thing here is nothing?" I couldn't believe it. "No. Nothing at all. Though if you don't like it for aesthetic reasons, we can make an appointment to have it removed." And all of a sudden, the inside of my head began to teem with flowers pink, purple, and blue.

31

I met her at university, in the cloisters of the Facultat de Filologia. I'd stopped in to read for a bit because it was the only place near my apartment that was quiet, deserted, and free. She was putting up flyers for a photography exhibition of her best work until that moment – she had just bought her first professional camera. She had it, though – a knack for wresting beauty from the world with nothing but a small toy camera. Not only that, but she made the rare kind of work that could set new parameters. Her pictures of Barcelona, Paris, and Normandy introduced novel ways of understanding photography; a constant recreation of spaces as real, pious, and intense as virgins, they injected the world with subtle innovations. The woman was Roxanne and she lived in an extraordinary and crazy totality that I was a part of for a while. As she worked, her whole being turned into this totality, which was what I found most attractive about her – that nuclear and groundbreaking intimacy that she could lay bare and sustain with her art, with her work. I know now that she was the first woman I ever loved. "Can I help?" I asked that morning. She looked at me, knowing exactly what would happen between us. Her nose, cheeks, and lips were a little pinched, as though annoyed and at the same amused by the ordinariness of the people with whom she was forced to coexist. I struck back with a smug

cock of the eyebrow and parting my lips in an expression
that used to drive my mother up the wall when I was a kid,
because who did I think I was going around with my nose
in the air, aged just ten or twelve or fifteen. The first time
I was hauled over the coals for it, I had no idea what she was
talking about. But after being repeatedly scolded, I finally
realized that the expression in question, which was really
just a demonstration of interest in something or someone,
might be seen as "having an attitude" with respect to other
people, especially grown-ups. "You think you're better than
everyone, don't you?" said Mom one Sunday at a restaurant,
after I had polished off my half-portions of escudella and
veal with mushrooms, gotten up from my seat, and headed
toward the bathroom across a roomful of tables overflowing
with plates and people in all shapes and sizes. There were
women with blonde perms stacked on their heads. This was
verboten at home, where hair was always worn straight
and natural with bangs like an oppressive helmet. Except
for Dad, of course. Men's hairdos are like Apple operating
systems, highly compatible with all forms of life. Next to the
door to the restroom was a table where a laid-back married
couple sat with their three grown children, two boys and
a girl. They chatted and laughed while sharing forkfuls of
food. Slender and long-limbed, their children were pure
lifeblood. The girl was stunning, her face made up in white
with two black lines across her eyes and garnet lips so dark
they were almost black, like All Souls' Day roses. I'd never
seen such impressive lips – velvety and full, a touch of red
sauce from the pastís de peix in the corner of her mouth,
enticing as candy. I didn't care for fish, but Mom could have
easily persuaded me to eat it with a girl like that. It can't
have taken me longer than two seconds to walk past her, but
that was enough to see the red highlights in her hair. Her

hair was fake and disheveled! I went into the bathroom and masturbated feverishly. I was only fifteen years old, with all of Sunday evening ahead of me. Eighteen seemed eons away. As I walked back to the table, I noticed that Mom looked more sour-faced than usual. "You think you're better than everyone, don't you?" "Where do you think you're going on that high horse?" That was Dad. Oh no. I looked over at my father. Had he been abducted? He never talked to me like that – actually, he never talked to me much at all, except to say "brush your teeth" and "goodnight." Mom wasn't to be trusted, but Dad . . . Dad filled me with doubt. That morning, I used the same expression on Roxanne, who smiled back. She had lovely teeth, pearly and upright like a row of novices.

32

I want another sister and I know how to get one. This desire for a new sister is sudden and intense. When a twelve-year-old wants something, that's all there is to it. Even a sister. I'm only now wondering why. Where had that longing come from? What void had produced it, or the need for what void? The fact is that my parents were always on my case – especially Mom – and it can be difficult to breathe with your mother squatting on your ribs. My sister and I are only a couple of years apart. She's in the same situation as I am, beneath me, bearing a comparable amount of weight. But a new sister . . . a new sister is like a whole new flank! I head straight to my parents' bedroom. It's a special bedroom, much more special than that of any old parents. Mom has a long history of depression and migraines and suffers from chronic insomnia. The upstairs neighbors, a grandma and grandpa, make life impossible for her with their slippers. Honest to God, wearing slippers like flip-flops is like walking around in tap shoes. Apparently they're always moving chairs around, too. "What the hell are they doing up there?" Mom cries out. "They're probably sweeping," Dad ventures. "Since when does it take forty-five minutes to sweep under the table?" Mom is beside herself and ends up sobbing. Dad can't take it anymore and goes out to buy soft-soled slippers, two pairs in small grandma and grandpa sizes, and felt pads for the chair feet. All with money from his own pocket. He pays Grandma and Grandpa a surprise visit, helps them into their slippers, and sticks a square of felt to every chair foot. I still have trouble imagining their conversation and the looks on the faces of those two golden-agers. A week of peace and tranquility follows. But Grandma and Grandpa aren't sold on their new slippers – the soles let in the chill – and unable to withstand the imperceptible yet constant erosion of every-day use, the felt pads come unstuck. The torture once again ensues. Mom is unstable and always resting. My sister and I receive strict orders from our father not to break the silence, under threat of being sent to boarding school. I am drawn to the idea of boarding school. I've devoured every book in the Puck series and want nothing more than to swap my house for a boarding school. The thought is so thrilling I convince my sister we should argue more than ever. But Dad doesn't make good on his threats and the blind trust I once had in him is lost. Dad has a lot of other qualities, though. He's got the makings of a secret agent or an inven-tor – he's highly adaptable and can bounce back with incred-ible ease. Not afraid to carry through even the wildest schemes, he cooks up a foolproof plan to turn the master bedroom into a soundproof suite. My sister and I can't believe it. The construction workers tear down the room and stuff it with foam and insulation materials of surprising textures, making it smaller. They pad *everything* – the walls, ceiling, floor, even the door and the insides of the built-in closets. An interior decorator then puts up wallpaper, leaving the walls taut and shiny like the inside of a jewelry box. Then come the power outlets, headboard, bed frame, mattress, nightstands, lamps, curtains, and dresser. A fitted carpet, too! Mom and Dad walk in without shoes on, but my sister and I are strictly forbidden from entering, which feels really unfair. Walking on that carpet must be the nicest thing in the world – it's beautiful, plush and green like grass. All it takes is seeing it from the doorway for me to feel the uncontainable urge to trample on it. But the carpet is made of these ruthless fucking fibers that imprint the exact size of the foot in a darker shade of green. I once tried to retrace Mom and Dad's footsteps, but even that failed: Inside theirs, my footprints were lighter. Darned carpet! Even snow is less treacherous. Mom found out that I had violated her sacred space and put me through an interrogation. Mom's interrogations are sociopathic; smooth and diabolical, they fill me with guilt. The woman knows how to crack open the door to your existential void, and her Mom-insults, though small, are enough to nudge you over the edge and send you tumbling down. All the same, today I am twelve years old and I've figured out a way around her intuitive sense of surveillance: plastic bags. Plastic bags! I had seen Mom using them to grab something from her bedroom on the quick when she was already wearing her outside shoes. She would pull a grocery bag over each shoe and skate over the carpet without leaving a trace. This afternoon, I follow suit. I slip a bag over one foot, then the other, and slide silently toward the closet as if over ice. On the third shelf on the left-hand side of the closet is the sewing kit, a sort of picnic basket with foam padding, a floral pattern, and ruffles around the lid. I place it on the bed, open the lid, and begin to rummage for a small case – not the one for pins but the one for sewing needles, which are much finer. Mom has always been very tidy, but the sewing kit is mayhem, a lair of measuring tapes and ribbons. My dreams are going to be crawling with snakes tonight. I set aside useless boxes full of buttons. Mom is an avid collector of buttons. Before getting rid of an old piece of clothing, she often makes a point to remove the buttons first. Why? It must be an innate scarcity mindset. She also collects rolls of Gutermann thread in every color. Most of them are new – she has a tendency to buy thread in the exact color of the clothing she has to mend, even when darning socks. I realize now that the unassuming sewing kit was actually a coffer, each roll of thread worth a small fortune. After a lot of poking around, I unearth a small tube of sewing needles from a morass of pairless socks and select the finest needle. I put the sewing kit back in its place, shut the closet door, and kneel at my dad's nightstand. My nerves are frayed. Rather, my nerves are a time-lapse of a plant growing from seed into a forest, the sudden and unexpected bloom of millions of shoots around my solar plexus. Bam! From zero to millions in a fraction of a second. I can feel my nerves rooting around for a space of their own, for some comfort, throwing up inside me a thicket of roots and trunks, of branches and litterfall. This is how I feel as I kneel at Dad's nightstand, at his small and sacred altar. They've got to be in there. I open the drawer. A line of white Abanderado underpants, folded up nice and neat just like my panties. I rifle through the three front rows and then feel around the rows of underpants in the back, which are probably older and more threadbare. It's almost the same as my underwear drawer, except the panties in the back of mine don't fit. Mom only keeps them for emergencies. I shut the drawer. Solid wood slides along tracks like a plea for silence and comes to a sudden stop. I open the two bottom doors, which remind me of a tabernacle with knobs like pendulous steel earrings. Inside is a heap of unidentifiable objects, and a very hard cardboard box with the word *Duward* printed in black on the lid, the edges worn and soft like the skin of an apricot. Inside, nothing. Behind the box, I feel pieces of paper, and right next to it an empty space that I sweep with my fingers. It seems strange that there should be empty space in such a small cupboard, but I don't care because in the back on the right-hand side, I find what I'm looking for: a small box in a plastic wrapper. When I touch it, the plastic crackles like it would on a package of cookies. I know I've found what I'm looking for before even taking it out. I hold it in one hand and study it in detail: a bright red box with the words *Durex* and *24 condoms*. My heart pounds like a fist. I open the box and pull out a metallic plastic sleeve printed with text. I've gotten my hands on Dad's condoms! They're right inside, two condoms separated by a dotted line, one on top and one on the bottom, like giant painkillers. I grab the needle and slowly pierce the sleeve, right through the middle, until the tip comes out the other side. There's a tiny but visible hole and I press the plastic with my finger until I can hardly see the incision. I swallow the saliva that has pooled in my mouth and move on to the next condom. Though I would like to put every condom in the box through the same procedure, I might get caught and these two should do the trick. I leave everything as it was and exit the bedroom. In the kitchen, I open the door to the cupboard that holds the trash can – at home, everything is carefully tucked away in cupboards – and thrust my hand into the garbage. As I feel around the trash for somewhere to stash the sewing needle and plastic bags, I come into contact with moist lunch scraps and pray there won't be a repeat of the time Mom lost her wedding ring. In the end, Dad had set up a kind of street vendor situation with newspapers lining the floor of the sunroom, pulled on dishwashing gloves, and went about extracting the rubbish in layers. Plastic encrusted with food scraps, damp paper towels, weird clumps, Mom's sanitary pads, and lunch spa-ghetti all mixed together. The spaghetti was mine. It was unsettling, like a documentary still of a small, partially digested seal in the stomach of a dead shark washed up on shore. But Dad was a champ. He worked in silence, his head clear and hands steady, but there was no sign of the ring, which showed up in a pocket of Mom's bathrobe days later. I'm worried that the same thing could happen today, now that I've dumped the bags and the needle in the trash. A needle may be your average, everyday object, but finding average, everyday objects where they don't belong is an obvious red flag. I tell myself it won't happen, that there's just no way it'll happen, and I recite the Lord's Prayer, a Hail Mary, the Creed, and the Beatitudes.

33

I left, and sometime later, Roxanne slit her wrists. She sliced them open like a fisherwoman would the belly of a sea bass, except the incisions she made were neat, exceptionally thin, and undramatic. For all that, they still got to her in time, and they still saved her. They filled her with blood donated by do-gooders who had made room in their thoughts for all kinds of people except those who would attempt suicide, then returned her to her family in Marseille. I learned about this later. And when I did, it dawned on me that Roxanne was the only woman I had ever left for the simple reason that I was made to feel subhuman in her company, like a plaster mold from which she cast a life of abundance, a life open to the world, as simple and elegant as a Courbet and of the same overwhelming beauty, as pure as a morning of blue skies. Bonjour, Mademoiselle Roxanne. Comment allez-vous? says the gleaner with hairy hands and strong back, my whole self a mass of blood rushing to the head, my nose webbed with throbbing spider veins, and my future a skull that I trample while burning fields of stubble. Roxanne's alabaster forearms storm into my memory at unlikely moments. When the wilted spray of primroses vanishes from the roundabouts overnight and in their place rise red- and white-headed tulips. When I go to the supermarket late on a Saturday and the meat freezers are cold, long, and empty, but still glowing with light. When a cloud moves and yet seems to go nowhere, as though inside it somebody was making love in secret. When I go for a swim in the pool and am the first to break the surface. The helplessness and levity, the emptiness and perfection of Roxanne and her forearms when they were still forearms without any trace of history.

34

December 30. It's half past eleven at night in the children's ward of Vall d'Hebron University Hospital. Ten days have passed since my six-year-old niece was admitted with acute anterior uveitis in both eyes. It started as a harmless case of conjunctivitis. The pediatrician said it was nothing and pre-scribed eye drops. Three days later, my niece's eyes were bloodshot, and she cried literal tears of blood – followed by absolute blindness. My sister spent every day at the hospital looking after the girl, with her three-month-old latched to her breast. I have no idea how she managed to live her life without medication through all the months of pregnancy and breastfeeding. Her husband the engineer was in Shanghai for work. He wouldn't be back for another three weeks. "Do you want me to tell you a story, Auntie?" asks my niece from her hospital bed. Her name is Clàudia and I found out three days ago that she is extraordinary. Shame about the parents. She's an exceptional girl with no choice but to grow under the dark dome of a bell jar. At first my sister refused to leave her side, but she soon ran out of strength. Hospitals being Mom's favorite place to go, she took over with gusto. She quit after two days. She was grateful for Clàudia but more grateful still for the Hästens horsehair mattress waiting for her at home. I stepped in as her replacement. I didn't sleep a wink that first night. The second night, my body took control and forced me to rest; it was sort of like an induced slumber, about as violent as a stoning. The third night marked the complete digestion of my self. The hospital absorbs into its perfect organism the body and what remains of the care-giver's soul, and the outside world is forgotten. If I crane my neck a little, I can see the beltway from the hospital room window. At night the cars look like comets driven by inscru-table mood swings. They appear this way, I think, because hospitals generate new levels of emotion that are more compassionate and nuanced. Clàudia is humanly flawless. Her main concern is to make sure I'm okay. She can't see a thing and her prognosis is uncertain; the ophthalmologists still haven't determined the cause of her blindness. They say it might be an infection or the result of some rheumatic disease. Apparently, eyes are like joints, susceptible to arthri-tis. On second thought, this isn't the least bit surprising. Eyes are excellent buffers, like elbows and knees. The doctors say they've sent samples of Clàudia's blood to the European Union in an attempt to put our minds at ease. I picture a building with an enormous depot of viruses and bacteria – a sort of bacterial library of restricted access – in some sterile location in Belgium or Germany. From the way they explain this to us, I realize that doctors believe the words "European Union" have magical properties capable of soothing the nerves of mothers and fathers, but it hasn't worked on me. On my third day, I put in a request for a couple of personal days and promise to work harder than ever from the play-room of the children's ward. There's no one there at night, a quiet space full of mutilated dolls with staring eyes. This pleases me; it makes my solitude feel relative. I've always thought of hospitals as welcoming, maybe because the staff are awake around the clock, guardians of the night who help people feel safe in their little bubbles. My sister stops by every morning and evening, almost always with Mom. Pale and with bags under her eyes, she's not so much white as discolored, her musculature gray and see-through. Mom, meanwhile, looks splendid. Her skin is radiant and her talking points inexhaustible. She is in her element at hospitals, a state of exception that's like a prelude to orgasm. My sister mentioned today that she's considering taking a course of antianxiety meds, except she might wait a while longer because the baby's still breastfeeding and she wants to be a good mom. I tell her that good and evil are relative in the face of an imperative like a mother's love. I tell her that children are tiny archives of unconditionality, and that love is an absolute, impervious to feeding methods. Her survival takes precedence over that of her children, or else it would be impossible for her to ensure their continued existence. But she isn't listening; she is convinced she's done something wrong and that her eldest is paying for it. Her guilt is obliterating. She hasn't eaten in days and her tear ducts are spent. I swear to every god that exists that I will never have kids. I swear it a hundred thousand times. I have to. A few days later, my sister has abandoned every pretense of a healthy lifestyle, as though it had only ever been a distraction, as though eco-friendly living had only ever offered a false sense of security. Having a daughter admitted to the hospital with absolute blindness is like an air-raid siren: All of a sudden life explodes violently in your head, magnifying its sense and absence in equal measure. I comfort her and promise to look after Clàudia until she is discharged. I pop home in the evening and stuff clothes, books, and a toiletry bag into a suitcase, then settle into an awful pleather armchair at Clàudia's bedside. She draws with her eyes shut and asks if she's doing a good job. She draws lilac trees laden with yellow apples that slip away from the branches and climb crookedly up to the sky. Her drawing is so beautiful it would make Van Gogh jealous, I say. When Clàudia laughs, she raises her face just like a girl who is definitively blind. I promise to keep her pictures safe until she can see them. Her smile makes hot, fat tears flow from my eyes, the ghosts of predecessors unknown and invincible that roll down my cheeks like blistering metal. I tell her I'm going to pop over to the bathroom, and then I cry. I cry all over myself, even though I don't want to and don't not want to. Hundreds of mothers have fallen to pieces in this bathroom, I think. But I'm not crying for Clàudia and I don't think I am crying for me, either. I weep like sugar from fruit left too long on a branch. I melt. I give in. I turn little by little into a sack of bones. After I have been in there too long, I wash my face and head back to Clàudia. She gropes my arm and slides her hand down until it meets mine and gives it a hard squeeze. "Don't cry, Auntie. Do you want the TV on?" I realize she's the only person in the world I can be honest with. "If you like, we can find some cartoons and I'll tell you what's happening," I say. It's a fun game because the cartoons move fast and I have to talk faster than usual. She pisses herself laughing. I apply three different eye drops to each eye every hour on the dot. Night and day. This is the nurses' job, but they were making mistakes, so I told them I would do it myself. I find it unnerving for Clàudia's pupils to be permanently dilated by eye drops and for her to not see a thing. She gazes out like a bewildered cat at night, uncomplaining. She only loses her composure when they come to take blood. She's terrified of needles and the nurse who draws her blood is a sadist. I've noticed that in general, the medical staff lie a lot. Not to grown-ups but to children, which makes for children who are terrified and completely untrusting. I insist that they tell her the truth. "Come on, just one more little prick and I'll be gone for good," says the sadist. She's lying. She'll be back to prick her two more times and then again tomorrow. "It doesn't hurt," they lie. Clàudia looks at me without seeing. She wants a truth to hold onto. "It's going to hurt a little, but then it'll pass. I'll be right here with you," I promise. The doctors look at me like I've gone mad. Clàudia screws up her face and screams as the needle breaks her skin and slowly enters her vein, but she keeps her arm steady with an impressive force of will as her small hand crushes the bones in mine. She later confesses that the hands of the nurse holding down her ankles had hurt even more than the needle. I hug her and she hugs me. I don't think I've ever felt so embraced. Clàudia puts her ear to my chest and listens to my heart, which is spurred by her to deepen its beat. A hard-rock lullaby grows inside me, cracking the permafrost. I break, and as I break the only thing I want to do is bury my face in Clàudia's hair, which is shiny and beautiful even under the fluorescent light. The next day, my sister comes alone, leaving Arlet in the waiting room with Mom. Mom is thrilled by the prospect of playing the role of grandma to a hospital audience, who are not a particularly demanding audience, sentenced as they are to a tedium worse than illness. My sister explains that she's started a twofold treatment of antianxiety meds and antidepressants. She's also on pills to suppress lactation. She says her breasts hurt and lifts them like we used to as kids pretending to be grown women with oranges under our shirts. Arlet is a cooperative baby and takes to the bottle without fuss. She digests the formula more slowly, so she also sleeps more, "which is helpful," my sister says. I observe the way she and Clàudia interact. The girl is protective, and every little thing my sister does is a thing she has learned from being a mother, and though she demonstrates infinite care for her daughter, it somehow remains inexplicably outside the realm of real communication. I want my sister to go home and leave me with Clàudia. Some wishes come from an intolerable place; they're as filthy as a shovelful of manure and just as nutritious. My sister looks up, thanks me, and leaves.

35

It's half past eleven on the night of January 5. I've decided that as soon as Clàudia gets her sight back, I am done. I won't waste another minute. I'll do it from my roof terrace. There's a small communal area below, and in the dead of winter the risk of crushing any innocent human creatures is nil; plus, the building is modern and therefore devoid of cats. I picture the impact, cubic and dense – the skull split open, thoughts flowing thick and lava-like along the pavement as they try to get away from me. I am an imperfect woman, stiff as licorice, flinty and exasperating as a splinter of rabbit bone wedged between two molars. I hope they find me before the birds spot my eyeballs. Birds have always inspired in me a sort of ancestral terror; their despotic beaks admit no feelings and I have feelings. Right now, I feel the quiet of a hand that enters my belly, the ensuing cramps, a sharp pain that grows to the size of a termite hill. I feel the termite hill inside me, a cloud of red and orange dust, a crypt about to walk off. I won't leave a note. I don't want to leave behind any trace of cruelty. Clàudia is a little better today. Her eyes seem to be responding to treatment. But it's an odd sort of treatment, an aggressive and crude blend of antibiotics and antirheumatics the doctors have pulled from their sleeves in a last-ditch effort. There's something biblical about it all. I experience a terror like the terror of the weeks preceding the obliteration of an entire town, but there's nothing I can do, so I just apply eye drops around the clock. Her eyes are now large mirrored wells that have started to spring leaks, drenching and neutralizing the hostile chemistry with sub-soil efficiency. When I look at her, I see a lake lost in its own depth, a lake black and crystal clear. She learns from it and I unlearn from her. I draw away and pace up and down spiral staircases that fill me and try to communicate something to me. I've realized that I know myself by heart – I know myself to the point of recognizing people who don't exist and yet complement me. I know myself like a path that leads home, like a doorless corridor, like endless guardrails. I know myself like a decade-long involuntary commitment. To end and be done with it. I sense a change in my body – it is unsexed, majestic and magnificently afflicted, like a tower riddled with sorrow. And I can feel the whole crush of humanity inside me, concentrated in a place that is absolutely personal.

36

Day 10. It's been three days since Clàudia was discharged. Yesterday my sister left both Clàudia and Arlet with our mom. Mom would have liked to only take care of the baby, but she looks after Clàudia by buying her favorite snack, a sweet pastry with pine nuts. The absolute helplessness of babies gives Mom a cruel sense of satisfaction – it's a hidden cruelty, present like the tiny minute hand on a watch. Clàudia has regained her eyesight completely. The swelling was so extensive her irises had cleaved to her lenses and left behind secret constellations in their own dark, quasi-black pigment, constellations that could only be detected in a dark room by an ophthalmologist with a lens like a small telescope. Meaning, Clàudia is doing well. I look at her and see a web of happiness hanging over her, an intrinsic silk, just as I'd observed when she was still blind. She's an odd girl; she reminds me of me, except the polar opposite. My sister has gone to collect her husband from the airport. He came back because it was time. People like my sister and brother-in-law can swallow anything, never mind if later on reality pierces them like a nail in the coralline wall of a stomach – they've got tentacles that can wrap around it to an unnatural degree, masking their misfortune. Sometimes it feels possible to do as they do, to live bloodlessly and gallop toward the yellow evening horizon, like a dead man tied to a stake.

37

Day 11. Today I've learned that death is transferable.

38

Day 14. Dad cries. Mom cries and a part of her cries out of spite. Arlet screams. Clàudia concentrates her pain in the palm of her hand and clutches mine as if her blood were still being drawn. The priest is a sadist who has the gall to say the word "resurrection," which is much worse than lying. I sink into something like my own private ocean. Joaquim and Cristina, I hear, model parents. Joaquim and Cristina, happily married. The girl who plays the violin has dark circles under her eyes from partying all night. The sound of the violin is proper, unfeeling, accommodating. Dad bows his head the way a man might bow his whole body. The room is fragrant with the green scent of stiff leaves and stiff, chilled flowers. The floor and its ancient bedrock of sorrow are covered in a thin layer of brightness. Sorrow is an enormous mystery light-years away from love, I think. The light is unreal. The windows are unreal. The people are a cluster of dresses and shoes. Arlet sucks on her pacifier with brute force, her stroller rocking faintly to the pulse of her rage. Clàudia looks at me and says Auntie. My sister has left her daughters in the care of their aunt. She's left them in *my* care. Even though I'm single, even though I'm gay, even though I'm suicidal. Auntie is a responsible person now. This morning, I made myself some fresh orange juice and washed it down with pills. I smile without crying. Smiling like this thaws the permafrost. The violin plays on. Families huddle like villages under siege. But the savagery that stalks and besieges us – is life.

A TRANSLATOR'S AFTERWORD

— *Pensez-vous que la poésie (la vôtre a fortiori) peut être traduite?*

— *Non, et pourtant elle l'est.*

ANNE CARSON, INTERVIEWED IN *LE DEVOIR*

Permafrost started as a prompt in a therapy session. "Write about your life," the author's therapist instructed, and Eva Baltasar obeyed. Before long she grew bored of the truth and began to inject fiction into her writing. She left therapy shortly after. This may be more anecdotal than it is revelatory, and yet it closes in on a quality I feel is integral to the text: its *searching*.

By the time *Permafrost* was first published in 2018, Eva Baltasar had written and published ten poetry collections. I think of Eva Baltasar first and foremost as a poet, and have always admired in her that curious impulsiveness I often attribute to poets. In her early twenties, for example, Eva moved to the mountains of Catalonia with her two-year-old daughter. Her nearest neighbor was a shepherd who lived three kilometers away. In exchange for milk and cheese, she helped the shepherd with his chores; she also used his washing machine. Meanwhile, she would write on the computers of her daughter's school. There is a similar impulsiveness at work in the way our protagonist navigates the world, always seeking to find a home for herself on the margins of a conventional life.

Translator and author Jennifer Croft once spoke of identifying the "heart" of a novel, and how this can become key to its translation. Like an octopus, I believe a novel has several hearts. Aside from its searching, one of the heart-keys to *Permafrost* may be in the novel's dedication: *To poetry, for permitting it.*

* * *

Marguerite Duras as translated by Olivia Baes and Emma Ramadan writes that "translation is not a matter of the literal exactitude of a text, but perhaps we must go even further: and say that it is more of a musical approach, rigorously personal and even, if necessary, deviant." I learned one day over lunch with Eva Baltasar's editor that her only condition during edits was that the word in question be replaced with one that was similarly stressed or unstressed, as the case may be. What mattered was how each word affected the *music* of the sentence, what this music conveyed, and how the music delivered up the image to the reader. An example:

> Catalan: Jo em sent*i*a cada d*i*a més empetit*i*da, redu*ï*da, a una c*o*rtineta de c*u*ina al seu c*o*stat.

> My translation: I felt smaller and smaller by the day, next to her nothing but a frilly kitchen curtain.

Let's look at the words in detail, or rather in musical detail. Hopefully my highlights have helped to make clear what's at play in this sentence. It may be odd to speak of a sentence being moved in a certain direction – we read from left to right in English, so what other direction could it possibly go? – and yet there is a definite sense here of being ushered forward by the end rhymes (ee-ah, ee-ah, ee-dah, ee-dah) of the first clause as they flow into the head rhymes of the second (coo, coo, coo), and come to a sudden and dry stop: co*stat.*

The image is a bit odd, or at least odd enough that it puzzled the English editor. One thing she wanted to know was: What *is* a kitchen curtain? Though the simile seemed obvious to me – "it's one of those ridiculously tiny curtains that are sheer and mostly decorative," I wrote in the comments – one thing I have learned from translating is that when an image is obvious to the translator but opaque to everyone else, there is often something missing. The fact that the editor had been puzzled by the image also raised several questions for me, all of which took me back to the dedication and helped inform the rest of my draft: Is it possible that the image owed its existence entirely to the musicality of the (Catalan) words? Had that felicitous, musical connection between the words *cortineta* and *cuina* not existed, would the author have arrived at this image at all? If so, what should I prioritize? Does the image take precedence over the music, or do I do my my best to maintain both? To what do I owe my contentious fidelity?

* * *

I keep returning to a phrase Duras uses in another essay of the same collection, when writing about her development as a writer. She writes: "It was with *Moderato Cantabile* . . . that I started to write – how should I put this – that I started to write nonsense in a given direction." This feels true to me about poetry, and about this poet's novel. Coupled with Duras' other observation about translation and music, I choose to read "given direction" as in the direction of music, focusing on sound and rhythm and on the sheer musical *materiality* of language.

* * *

I've had to take a different approach in my translation of the kitchen curtain sentence, of course, and I'd like to zoom in on a small Durassian deviation: the word *frilly*. It may surprise you to find out there are no frills on the Catalan kitchen curtain. What "frilly" seeks to capture instead is a close reading of the simile, and especially a close reading of the diminutive, *cortineta*. As any Romance speaker knows intuitively, the diminutive inserts a variety of nuances into a word, ranging from smallness to tenderness, and to depreciation, not all of which can be captured by "little," or "small," or "wee." The Catalan not only makes (a very natural) use of the diminutive, but also doubles down on the sense of demotion with the words "empetitida" and "reduïda." I have tried to reflect this in the English version by creating a sense of progressive reduction in "smaller and smaller" and finally in the "nothing but" in order to give the reader the feeling – much like the sentence's abrupt end with the word "costat" – that this is as small as our protagonist is able to feel in relation to the other character.

* * *

In a virtual lecture given at UMass just as the pandemic was beginning to send people into isolation, Jennifer Croft stated that what she wanted "to argue, ultimately, is that everything is indeed untranslatable if what translation is is making something new that stays the same. But that's not what translation is." When I think of discussions surrounding translation – of its possibility or impossibility – I often wonder whether the issue is not purely semantic, rather than practical. Would translation be quite so controversial if we were to simply call it something else? Would people still enter a translated text with as much suspicion if we called our little art something like "versioning" or "againing"? I am thinking of Kate Briggs when she writes: "Some new thing starts to get made in the frame of againness; something that is *of the original*, yes, but that will extend beyond the reach of it, the purview of it, since it is being made by someone else, by me now, and will be read, perhaps, by some or many others, all of them to come and for the moment elsewhere."

I often think of translation as a "craft" in the sense of "a branch of skilled work." "Craft" also contains a slew of other meanings, some of which are now technically obsolete and yet continue to haunt contemporary use of the word (a personal favorite is: "human skill, *art* as opposed to *nature*.") And because of who I am, when I think of craft, I think of ceramics. Of the original as the first vessel the artist creates and which they – and often others – recreate with the raw material available to them. Bear with me; this is not a perfect analogy. I am not a ceramic artist, but a translator who makes pots; I am not an author, but a writer who makes translations. What I am trying to get at is that the raw material used in ceramics – clay – is by nature hyperlocal and that the potter is singular: no handcrafted piece is ever the same, because its making is a process that takes place across time and in a space subject to the whims of the weather (salinity, humidity, dryness), of the firing method.

John, the potter who runs the studio where I make ceramics, likes to remind us that with every vessel we create, we are entering something new into the world that cannot be completely destroyed, which calls to mind a line in Johannes

Göransson's *Transgressive Circulation*: "The danger of translation is not just that it makes the original yet another version, but that it infects the entire literary culture with a proliferation of versions." I don't imagine that John is trying to dissuade us from making, from experimenting, from bringing our strange little vessels into the world. He is simply alerting us to the existence of a responsibility. And this thought rests at the back of my mind as I translate.

*   *   *

Another beating heart in *Permafrost* is its carnality, the way it depicts a body moving through and against the world. The world outside the body, with its demands for a certain behavior, and the world inside – not only on the level of thought but of bodily function – are in constant conflict throughout. The result is an intensity of feeling, something the protagonist both craves and balks at. Hence the permafrost, the thick layer of ice she's thrown up to protect her inner life from the living that's happening outside. Hence her fixation on sex, which allows her to safely bridge the two. Yet, if there is a conflict between the external and the internal, between thought and body, body and world, there is none around the objects of the body's desire.

In *Permafrost,* Eva Baltasar takes up issues that are often treated with kid gloves – a child's understanding of sex, death by suicide, illness – and addresses them with the same transparency due to anything else. She takes suicide seriously – there is always the danger that her protagonist will succeed – while finding humor in its physicality. As the protagonist prepares for the third suicide attempt of the novel, in the bathroom of her apartment, she wonders what will happen to her sphincters after she dies. Will they relax? Will she pee herself? Should she hedge her bets by giving herself an enema? By looking closely at the body and looking at its functions in painstaking detail, the author divests it of any real dignity or preciousness. It's just a body after all, and we have as little control over it as we do over anything else. Later in the novel, after the protagonist as child watches a porno with her friends for the first time and goes home to find that there is a sticky substance in her panties, she masturbates just like she does every day and finds herself thinking about her classmate Laura. The fact that she is a ten- or maybe eleven-year-old girl desiring a ten- or maybe eleven-year-old girl is a non-issue. And the fact that it's a non-issue, the naturalness of it, is another heart-key.

Which brings me to the word "cunt."

The first entry in the *Oxford English Dictionary* defines it as "the female genitals; the vulva or vagina." The next entry includes the words "promiscuous," "slut," "sexual gratification." It is also a general term of abuse for a woman – and for a man, notes the dictionary. In my experience, "cunt" is one of those pesky words that can split a room. Especially in the United States, where I have seen some of my most sexually forthcoming friends squirm at the sound of the plosive. It provokes a gut reaction. The Catalan equivalent, "cony" – whose etymological root is in the Latin for vulva, "cŭnnus" (see "cunnilingus") – is not so contentious. A general rule of mine when translating is to try to find words that occupy similar semantic spaces as the original. In this case, I'm not sure "cony" and "cunt" operate in quite the same way. "Cony" is more acrobatic in Catalan than the English word "cunt," which seems to have been delegated to the lexical margins. Merriam-Webster won't even give me synonyms; neither does Lexico, the site that uses the Oxford dictionary. Thesaurus.com gives me the following for "vagina or woman (used offensively)" in this order: bitch, pussy, beaver, box, cherry, clit, muff, puss, snatch, twat, gash, merkin, pudenda, slit, slut, vagina, and vulva, in that order. Some make me cringe (gash, slit), others make me laugh (merkin, muff), but in reality "pussy" seems like the only feasible alternative. Except, it's 2020, and Donald Trump has been President of the United States for nearly four years, and I can't help thinking of *that time* he said "pussy" and still won the election. "Cunt" may not occupy exactly the same semantic space as "cony" but it feels in line with the spirit of the book, with the naturalness of the author's treatment of the sexual body. In translating "cony" as "cunt" repeatedly and always inoffensively in these pages, I have striven to make it as much of a non-issue as desire is in *Permafrost*.

* * *

I'm sure I'm not the first person to think of the original text as a fraction of a whole. Picture a sphere. Picture the moon, even. When the reader directs their attention to a text as it exists in a single language, they are seeing only one face(t) of it, much like we only ever see one side of the moon from our singular viewpoint. The rest exists behind it, in darkness. Perhaps we can only participate in the full potential of any literary text once we have read it in every language and across all time. Maybe it's not translation that is impossible but rather a complete understanding of any piece of literature.

* * *

By the time this book is published, it will have been two years since Eva and I met for lunch at an Italian restaurant in Barcelona, where I wrote the first version of this translation in the rather bourgeois reading rooms of the Ateneu Barcelonès, with its checkered ceramic floors and leather desks. I used to sit with my laptop in front of me and stacks of English-language poetry and prose on either side, anchors that kept me from drifting too far into Catalan waters. Whenever I felt bested by a sentence, I'd gaze out the window into the paved courtyard shaded by tall palms and loud with birdsong, pick up one of the books I'd brought and let its English wash over me. I arrived at lunch with Eva armed with some of the books I'd been reading to inform my translation. Books of prose poetry (*Bluets, My Private Property*), long-form prose written by poets (*The Undying*), poetry tout court, *Good Morning, Midnight* by Jean Rhys, Anaïs Nin's diaries, Anne Carson. There were more, too. All of them by women. As I look back, I feel a little embarrassed about the fact that I did this; it's possible I felt these texts would give my work credence, in her eyes, or maybe I believed they had the power to show her I knew whose company I was bringing her into. She was confused, and I probably changed the subject to something else in the hope of distracting her. Over lunch, we shared tiramisu, her daughter's favorite dessert, and she was disappointed to find that they had made it with Nutella.

Perhaps translation is as much about being a careful reader and about having a good ear as it is about the details that settle like sand on the seabed of our memories, about the company we choose to keep, and about the place and the moment in time when we go about our craft – word by painstaking word.

JULIA SANCHES

PROVIDENCE, RHODE ISLAND, AUGUST 2020

Dear readers,

As well as relying on bookshop sales, And Other Stories relies on subscriptions from people like you for many of our books, whose stories other publishers often consider too risky to take on.

Our subscribers don't just make the books physically happen. They also help us approach booksellers, because we can demonstrate that our books already have readers and fans. And they give us the security to publish in line with our values, which are collaborative, imaginative and 'shamelessly literary'.

All of our subscribers:

- receive a first-edition copy of each of the books they subscribe to
- are thanked by name at the end of our subscriber-supported books
- receive little extras from us by way of thank you, for example: postcards created by our authors

BECOME A SUBSCRIBER, OR GIVE A SUBSCRIPTION TO A FRIEND

Visit andotherstories.org/subscriptions to help make our books happen. You can subscribe to books we're in the process of making. To purchase books we have already published, we urge you to support your local or favourite bookshop and order directly from them – the often unsung heroes of publishing.

OTHER WAYS TO GET INVOLVED

If you'd like to know about upcoming events and reading groups (our foreign-language reading groups help us choose books to publish, for example) you can:

- join our mailing list at: andotherstories.org
- follow us on Twitter: @andothertweets
- join us on Facebook: facebook.com/AndOtherStoriesBooks
- admire our books on Instagram: @andotherpics
- follow our blog: andotherstories.org/ampersand

This book was made possible thanks to the support of:

Aaron McEnery
Aaron Schneider
Abigail Walton
Adam Lenson
Adrian Astur Alvarez
Adrian Perez
Adriana Diaz Enciso
Aifric Campbell
Ailsa Peate
Aisha McLean
Ajay Sharma
Alan Donnelly
Alan Stoskopf
Alastair Gillespie
Alastair Whitson
Alecia Marshall
Alex Hoffman
Alex Lockwood
Alex Pearce
Alex Ramsey
Alex Robertson
Alexander Barbour
Alexander Leggatt
Alexandra Stewart
Alexandra Stewart
Alexandra Tilden
Ali Riley
Ali Smith
Ali Usman
Alice Morgan
Alice Shumate
Alice Smith
Alice Toulmin
Alice Tranah
Alice Wilkinson
Alison Hardy
Alison Layland
Alison Winston
Aliya Rashid
Alyse Ceirante
Alyssa Rinaldi
Alyssa Tauber

Amado Floresca
Amaia Gabantxo
Amalia Gladhart
Amanda
Amanda Astley
Amanda Dalton
Amanda Geenen
Amanda Maria
    Izquierdo
    Gonzalez
Amanda Read
Amber Da
Amelia Lowe
Amy Bessent
Amy Koheeallee
Andra Dusu
Andrea Barlien
Andrea Reece
Andrew Kerr-Jarrett
Andrew Lees
Andrew Marston
Andrew McCallum
Andrew Rego
Andy Corsham
Andy Marshall
Angelica Ribichini
Angus Walker
Ann Menzies
Anna-Maria Aurich
Anna Dowrick
Anna Gibson
Anna Milsom
Anna Zaranko
Anne Barnes
Anne Carus
Anne Boileau Clarke
Anne Craven
Anne Guest
Anne Kangley
Anne Magnier-Redon
Anne-Marie Renshaw
Anne Sticksel

Anne Willborn
Anonymous
Anonymous
Anonymous
Anthony Brown
Anthony Cotton
Anthony Quinn
Antoni Centofanti
Antonia Lloyd-Jones
Antonia Saske
Antony Pearce
Aoife Boyd
Archie Davies
Arthur John Rowles
Asako Serizawa
Ashleigh Sutton
Ashley Cairns
Audrey Mash
Audrey Small
Barbara Bettsworth
Barbara Mellor
Barbara Robinson
Barbara Spicer
Barbara Wheatley
Barry John Fletcher
Barry Norton
Barry Watkinson
Bart Van Overmeire
Ben Schofield
Ben Schroder
Ben Sharratt
Ben Thornton
Ben Walter
Ben Wormald
Benjamin Judge
Benjamin Pester
Bethlehem Attfield
Beverley Thomas
Bhakti Gajjar
Bianca Duec
Bianca Jackson
Bianca Winter

Bill Fletcher
Bjørnar Djupevik
  Hagen
Brendan Monroe
Briallen Hopper
Brian Anderson
Brian Byrne
Brian Smith
Brigita Ptackova
Briony Hey
Burkhard Fehsenfeld
Caitlin Halpern
Caitriona Lally
Cal Smith
Cam Scott
Cameron Adams
Camilla Imperiali
Campbell McEwan
Carla Ballin
Carla Castanos
Carol Mavor
Carolina Pineiro
Caroline Jupp
Caroline West
Cassidy Hughes
Catharine
  Braithwaite
Catherine Barton
Catherine Fearns
Catherine Lambert
Catherine
  Williamson
Catie Kosinski
Catriona Gibbs
Cecilia Cerrini
Cecilia Rossi
Cecilia Uribe
Ceri Webb
Chantal Wright
Charlene Huggins
Charles Fernyhough
Charles Kovach
Charles Dee Mitchell
Charles Raby

Charles Tocock
Charlie Cook
Charlotte Briggs
Charlotte Coulthard
Charlotte Middleton
Charlotte Stoneley
Charlotte Whittle
Charlotte Woodford
Chelsey Johnson
Cherilyn Elston
Cherise Wolas
China Miéville
Chloe Baird
Chris Blackmore
Chris Gostick
Chris Gribble
Chris Holmes
Chris Köpruner
Chris Lintott
Chris Potts
Chris & Kathleen
  Repper-Day
Chris Stevenson
Christian
  Schuhmann
Christina Moutsou
Christine Bartels
Christine Elliott
Christine and Nigel
  Wycherley
Christopher Allen
Christopher Homfray
Christopher Jenkin
Christopher Stout
Ciara Ní Riain
Claire Adams
Claire Adams
Claire Brooksby
Claire Hayward
Claire Potter
Clare Young
Clarice Borges
Clarissa Pattern
Clive Bellingham

Cody Copeland
Colin Denyer
Colin Matthews
Colin Hewlett
Collin Brooke
Cornelia Svedman
Cortina Butler
Courtney Lilly
Craig Kennedy
Csilla Toldy
Cynthia De La Torre
Cyrus Massoudi
Daisy Savage
Dale Wisely
Dana Behrman
Dana Lapidot
Daniel Coxon
Daniel Gillespie
Daniel Hahn
Daniel Jàrmai
Daniel Jones
Daniel Oudshoorn
Daniel Raper
Daniel Stewart
Daniel Wood
Daniela Steierberg
Danny Millum
Darina Brejtrova
Darren Davies
Dave Lander
David Anderson
David Coates
David Cowan
David Gould
David Greenlaw
David Hebblethwaite
David Higgins
David Hodges
David Johnson-
  Davies
David Kendall
David Key
David Leverington
David F Long

David McIntyre
David Miller
David Miller
David Reid
David Richardson
David Shriver
David Smith
David Thornton
Davis MacMillan
Dawn Bass
Dean Taucher
Debbie Pinfold
Deborah Banks
Declan Gardner
Declan O'Driscoll
Deirdre Nic
   Mhathuna
Denis Larose
Denis Stillewagt &
   Anca Fronescu
Denton Djurasevich
Detta Eldor
Diana Digges
Diane Humphries
Diane Salisbury
Dinesh Prasad
Dipika Mummery
Dirk Hanson
Dominic Nolan
Dominick Santa
   Cattarina
Dominique Brocard
Drew Gummerson
Duncan Clubb
Duncan Macgregor
Duncan Marks
Dustin Haviv
Dyanne Prinsen
Earl James
Ebba Aquila
Ebba Tornérhielm
Ed Tronick
Ekaterina Beliakova
Elaine Kennedy

Eleanor Maier
Eleanor Updegraff
Elena Galindo
Elif Aganoglu
Elina Zicmane
Elisabeth Cook
Elizabeth Braswell
Elizabeth Dillon
Elizabeth Draper
Elizabeth Franz
Elizabeth Guss
Elizabeth Leach
Elizabeth Perry
Elizabeth Seal
Ellen Beardsworth
Ellen Casey
Emeline Morin
Emily Armitage
Emily McCarthy
Emily Webber
Emma Barraclough
Emma Bielecki
Emma Louise Grove
Emma Morgan
Emma Page
Emma Patel
Emma Post
Ena Lee
Eric Anderson
Eric Cassells
Eric Reinders
Eric Tucker
Erin Cameron Allen
Esmée de Heer
Etta Searle
Eugene O'Hare
Eva Mitchell
Eva Oddo
Eve Corcoran
Ewan Tant
F Gary Knapp
Fay Barrett
Felix Valdivieso
Finbarr Farragher

Finn Williamson
Fiona Davenport
   White
Fiona Liddle
Fiona Mozley
Florian Duijsens
Forrest Pelsue
Fran Sanderson
Frances
   Christodoulou
Frances Spangler
Frances Thiessen
Francesca Brooks
Francesca Rhydderch
Francis Mathias
Frank van Orsouw
Frankie Mullin
Freddie Radford
Freya Killilea-Clark
Friederike Knabe
Gabriel Colnic
Gabriel and Mary de
   Courcy Cooney
Gabriel Martinez
Gareth Tulip
Gary Gorton
Gavin Smith
Gawain Espley
Gemma Bird
Genaro Palomo Jr
Geoff Thrower
Geoffrey Cohen
Geoffrey Urland
George Stanbury
Georgia Shomidie
Georgina Hildick-
   Smith
Georgina Norton
Gerry Craddock
Gill Boag-Munroe
Gillian Grant
Gillian Spencer
Gordon Cameron
Gosia Pennar

Graham Blenkinsop
Graham R Foster
Grant Rintoul
Hadil Balzan
Hamish Russell
Hanna Randall
Hanna Varady &
  Mikael Awake
Hannah Freeman
Hannah Jane
  Lownsbrough
Hannah Mayblin
Hannah Procter
Hannah Rapley
Hannah Vidmark
Hanora Bagnell
Hans Lazda
Harriet Stiles
Harriet Wade
Haydon Spenceley
Heather & Andrew
  Ordover
Heidi Gilhooly
Helen Brady
Helen Coombes
Helen Moor
Helena Buffery
Henriette
  Magerstaedt
Henrike
  Laehnemann
Henry Bell
Henry Patino
Hilary Barry
Holly Barker
Holly Down
Howard Robinson
Hugh Shipley
Hyoung-Won Park
Iain Forsyth
Ian Hagues
Ian McMillan
Ian Mond
Ian Whitfield

Ida Grochowska
Ifer Moore
Ilona Abb
Ingunn Vallumroed
Irene Croal
Irene Mansfield
Irina Tzanova
Isabel Adey
Isabella Garment
Isabella Weibrecht
Isabelle Schneider
Isobel Foxford
Izabela Jamrozik
J Drew Hancock-Teed
Jacinta Perez Gavilan
  Torres
Jack Brown
Jacob Blizard
Jacqueline Lademann
Jacqueline Ting Lin
Jacqui Hudson
Jacqui Jackson
Jade Yiu
Jadie Lee
Jake Baldwinson
James Avery
James Beck
James Crossley
James Cubbon
James Dahm
James Kinsley
James Lee
James Lehmann
James Lesniak
James Leveque
James Mewis
James Norman
James Portlock
James Scudamore
Jamie Cox
Jamie Mollart
Jamie Walsh
Jan Hicks
Jan Phillips

Jane Bryce
Jane Dolman
Jane Fairweather
Jane Leuchter
Jane Roberts
Jane Roberts
Jane Woollard
Janet Kofi-Tsekpo
Jasmine Gideon
Jason Grunebaum
Jason Lever
Jason Sim
Jason Timermanis
Jayne Watson
Jeff Collins
Jenifer Logie
Jennifer Arnold
Jennifer Fisher
Jennifer Higgins
Jennifer Mills
Jennifer Watts
Jenny Barlow
Jenny Huth
Jenny Newton
Jeremy Koenig
Jeremy Morton
Jeremy Wellens
Jerry Simcock
Jess Hazlewood
Jesse Coleman
Jesse Hara
Jesse Thayre
Jessica Cooper
Jessica Laine
Jessica Martin
Jessica Queree
Jessica Weetch
Jethro Soutar
Jill Harrison
Jo Harding
Joanna Luloff
Joanne Smith
Joao Pedro Bragatti
  Winckler

JoDee Brandon
Jodie Adams
Jody Kennedy
Joe Catling
Joe Gill
Joe Bratcher
Joel Swerdlow
Johannes Holmqvist
Johannes Menzel
John Bennett
John Berube
John Bogg
John Carnahan
John Conway
John Down
John Gent
John Hanson
John Higginson
John Hodgson
John Kelly
John Royley
John Shaw
John Steigerwald
John Winkelman
Jon Riches
Jon Talbot
Jonathan Blaney
Jonathan Fiedler
Jonathan Huston
Jonathan Paterson
Jonathan Ruppin
Jonathan Watkiss
Jonny Kiehlmann
Jose Machado
Joseph Camilleri
Joseph Darlington
Joseph Flading
Joseph Novak
Joseph Schreiber
Josh Calvo
Josh Sumner
Joshua Davis
Joshua McNamara
Joy Paul

Judith Austin
Judith Gruet-Kaye
Julia Shmotkina
Julia Harkey
    D'Angelo
Julia Von Dem
    Knesebeck
Julian Molina
Julie Greenwalt
Julienne van Loon
Juliet Birkbeck
Juliet and Nick
    Davies
Juliet Swann
Juraj Janik
Justine Goodchild
K Elkes
Kaarina Hollo
Kaelyn Davis
Karl Kleinknecht &
    Monika Motylinska
Kasper Haakansson
Kat Côté
Kate Attwooll
Kate Beswick
Kate Procter
Kate Shires
Katharine Freeman
Katharine Robbins
Katherine
    Mackinnon
Kathryn Dawson
Kathryn Edwards
Kathryn Hemmann
Kathryn Oliver
Kathryn Williams
Katia Wengraf
Katie Brown
Katie Kennedy
Katie Kline
Katie Grant
Katie Smart
Katy Robinson
Katy West

Keith Walker
Kennedy McCullough
Kenneth Blythe
Kenneth Michaels
Kent McKernan
Kerry Parke
Kieran Rollin
Kieron James
Kim Metcalf
Kira Josefsson
Kirsten Hey
Kirsten Ward
Kirsty Doole
Klara Rešetič
Kris Ann Trimis
Kristen Tcherneshoff
Krystale Tremblay-
    Moll
Krystine Phelps
Kysanna Shawney
Lacy Wolfe
Lana Selby
Laura Clarke
Laura Ling
Laura Rangeley
Laura Zederkof
Laura Batatota
Lauren Pout
Laurence Laluyaux
Laurie Sheck & Jim
    Peck
Laury Leite
Leanne Radojkovich
Lee Harbour
Leon Geis
Leonora Randall
Liliana Lobato
Lily Blacksell
Lily Hersov
Lily Robert-Foley
Lily Susan Todd
Linda Jones
Lindsay Attree
Lindsay Brammer

Lindsey Ford
Lindsey Harbour
Linette Arthurton
  Bruno
Lisa Agostini
Lisa Dillman
Lisa Fransson
Lisa Leahigh
Lisa Simpson
Lisa Weizenegger
Liz Clifford
Liz Ketch
Lorna Bleach
Lorna Scott Fox
Lottie Smith
Louise Evans
Louise Greenberg
Louise Hoelscher
Louise Smith
Luc Verstraete
Lucas J Medeiros
Lucia Rotheray
Lucile Lesage
Lucy Beevor
Lucy Gorman
Lucy Greaves
Lucy Moffatt
Ludmilla Jordanova
Luise von Flotow
Luke Loftiss
Lydia Trethewey
Lynda Graham
Lynn Fung
Lynn Martin
Lynn Ross
M Manfre
Madeline Teevan
Mads Pihl
  Rasmussen
Maeve Lambe
Magdaline Rohweder
Maggie Kerkman
Mahan L Ellison & K
  Ashley Dickson

Malgorzata Rokicka
Mandy Wight
Marcel Schlamowitz
Margaret Dillow
Maria Ahnhem
  Farrar
Maria Hill
Maria Lomunno
Maria Losada
Maria Pia Tissot
Marie Cloutier
Marie Donnelly
Marijana Rimac
Marina Castledine
Marina Galanti
Mario Sifuentez
Marisa Wilson
Marja S Laaksonen
Mark Harris
Mark Huband
Mark Sargent
Mark Scott
Mark Sheets
Mark Sztyber
Mark Waters
Marlene Adkins
Marlene Simoes
Martha Nicholson
Martha Stevns
Martin Brown
Martin Nathan
Mary Byrne
Mary Heiss
Mary Nash
Mary Wang
Mary Ellen Nagle
Mathias Ruthner
Mathilde Pascal
Matt Davies
Matt Greene
Matt O'Connor
Matteo Besana
Matthew Adamson
Matthew Armstrong

Matthew Black
Matthew Francis
Matthew Gill
Matthew Lowe
Matthew Warshauer
Matthew Woodman
Maureen Cullen
Maureen Pritchard
Max Cairnduff
Max Garrone
Max Longman
Max McCabe
Maya Chung
Meaghan Delahunt
Meg Lovelock
Megan Taylor
Megan Wittling
Meghan Goodeve
Melissa Beck
Melissa Quignon-
  Finch
Melissa Stogsdill
Meredith Jones
Meredith Martin
Michael Bichko
Michael Dodd
Michael James
  Eastwood
Michael Friddle
Michael Gavin
Michael Holt
Michael Kuhn
Michael Pollak
Michael Roess
Michael
  Schneiderman
Miguel Head
Mike Turner
Mildred Nicotera
Miles Smith-Morris
Miranda Gold
Miriam McBride
Molly Foster
Mona Arshi

Moray Teale
Morven Dooner
Muireann Maguire
Myka Tucker-
   Abramson
Myles Nolan
N Tsolak
Nan Craig
Nancy Jacobson
Nancy Oakes
Naomi Morauf
Naomi Sparks
Natalie Ricks
Nathalie Atkinson
Nathalie
   Karagiannis
Nathan McNamara
Nathan Weida
Neferti Tadiar
Nguyen Phan
Nicholas Brown
Nicholas Jowett
Nicholas Smith
Nick Chapman
Nick James
Nick Nelson &
   Rachel Eley
Nick Sidwell
Nick Twemlow
Nicola Hart
Nicola Mira
Nicola Sandiford
Nicola Scott
Nicole Matteini
Nicoletta Asciuto
Nigel Fishburn
Niki Sammut
Nikki Dudley
Nina Alexandersen
Nora Hart
Odilia Corneth
Olga Alexandru
Olga Zilberbourg
Olivia Payne

Órla Ní Chuilleanáin
   and Dónall Ó
   Ceallaigh
Pamela Tao
Patrick Hawley
Patrick Hoare
Patrick McGuinness
Paul Brackenridge
Paul Cray
Paul Daintry
Paul Jones
Paul Munday
Paul Robinson
Paul Scott
Paula Edwards
Paula Turner
Pauline
   Westerbarkey
Pavlos Stavropoulos
Penelope Hewett
   Brown
Perlita Payne
Peter Edwards
Peter Hudson
Peter McBain
Peter McCambridge
Peter Rowland
Peter Taplin
Peter Wells
Petra Stapp
Philip Herbert
Philip Warren
Philip Williams
Philipp Jarke
Phillipa Clements
Phoebe McKenzie
Phoebe Millerwhite
Piet Van Bockstal
PRAH Foundation
Prakash Nayak
Priya Sharma
Rachael de Moravia
Rachael Williams
Rachel Carter

Rachel Dolan
Rachel Matheson
Rachel Meacock
Rachel Van Riel
Rachel Watkins
Rachel Watkins
Rebecca Braun
Rebecca Carter
Rebecca
   Micklewright
Rebecca Moss
Rebecca O'Reilly
Rebecca Parry
Rebecca Peer
Rebecca Roadman
Rebecca Rose
Rebecca Rosenthal
Rebecca Shaak
Rebekka Bremmer
Rhiannon Armstrong
Rhodri Jones
Rich Sutherland
Richard Ashcroft
Richard Catty
Richard Ellis
Richard Gwyn
Richard Harrison
Richard Mansell
Richard Priest
Richard Sanders
Richard Shea
Richard Soundy
Rick Tucker
Rita O'Brien
Robert Gillett
Robert Hamilton
Robert Hannah
Robin Taylor
Robina Franko
Rogelio Pardo
Roger Newton
Roger Ramsden
Ronan Cormacain
Rory Williamson

Ros Woolner
Rosalind May
Rosalind Ramsay
Rosanna Foster
Rose Crichton
Roxanne O'Del
    Ablett
Roz Simpson
Rupert Ziziros
Ruth Deyermond
Ryan Day
S Italiano
Sabine Little
Sally Baker
Sally Bramley
Sally Hall
Sally Hemsley
Sam Gordon
Sam Reese
Sam Southwood
Samantha Cox
Samuel Crosby
Samuel Wright
Sara Nesbitt Gibbons
Sara Kittleson
Sara Quiroz
Sara Sherwood
Sarah Allman
Sarah Arboleda
Sarah Elizabeth
Sarah Farley
Sarah Forster
Sarah Lucas
Sarah Manvel
Sarah Pybus
Sarah Roff
Sarah Spitz
Scott Astrada
Scott Chiddister
Scott Russell
Sean McDonagh
Sez Kiss
Shannon Knapp
Sharon Dogar

Sharon McCammon
Shauna Gilligan
Shauna Rogers
Sheila Duffy
Sheila Packa
Sheryl Jermyn
Shira Lob
Shona Holmes
Sian Hannah
Sienna Kang
Simon Clark
Simon Gray
Simon Pitney
Simon Robertson
Simonette Foletti
SK Grout
Sophia Wickham
ST Dabbagh
Stacy Rodgers
Stefanie Schrank
Stefano Mula
Stephan Eggum
Stephanie Lacava
Stephanie Shields
Stephanie Laurindo
    Da Silva
Stephen Cunliffe
Stephen Pearsall
Steve Chapman
Steve James
Steve Raby
Steven & Gitte Evans
Steven Vass
Steven Willborn
Stu Hennigan
Stuart Grey
Stuart Snelson
Stuart Wilkinson
Subhashree Beeman
Susan Bates
Susan Edsall
Susan Ferguson
Susan Winter
Susie Sell

Suzanne Kirkham
Sylvie Zannier-Betts
Tamara Larsen
Tamsin Walker
Tania Hershman
Tara Pahari
Tara Roman
Tasmin Maitland
Taylor Ffitch
Teresa Werner
Teri Hoskin
The Mighty Douche
    Softball Team
Thom Cuell
Thom Keep
Thomas van den
    Bout
Thomas Fritz
Thomas Mitchell
Thomas Smith
Thomas Andrew
    White
Tian Zheng
Tiffany Lehr
Tim Kelly
Tim Scott
Tim Theroux
Timothy Cummins
Tina Rotherham-
    Winqvist
Toby Halsey
Toby Ryan
Tom Darby
Tom Doyle
Tom Franklin
Tom Gray
Tom Stafford
Tom Whatmore
Tony Bastow
Tory Jeffay
Tracy Bauld
Tracy Heuring
Tracy Lee-Newman
Trevor Wald

Tricia Durdey
Tricia Pillay
Val Challen
Valerie O'Riordan
Vanessa Baird
Vanessa Dodd
Vanessa Fuller
Vanessa Heggie
Vanessa Nolan
Vanessa Rush
Victor Meadowcroft
Victoria Eld

Victoria Goodbody
Victoria Huggins
Victoria Maitland
Vijay Pattisapu
Wendy Langridge
William
  Brockenborough
William Dennehy
William Franklin
William Richard
William Schwaber
William Wood

Xanthe Rendall
Yaseen Khan
Yasmin Alam
Yoora Yi Tenen
Zachary Hope
Zara Rahman
Zezinha De Senha
Zoe Taylor
Zoe Thomas
Zoë Brasier

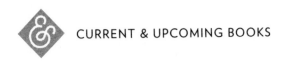

CURRENT & UPCOMING BOOKS

EVA BALTASAR has published ten volumes of poetry to widespread acclaim. Her debut novel, *Permafrost*, received the 2018 Premi Llibreter from Catalan booksellers and is short-listed for France's 2020 Prix Médicis for Best Foreign Book. It is the first novel in a triptych which aims to explore the universes of three different women in the first person. The author lives a simple life with her wife and two daughters in a village near the mountains.

JULIA SANCHES translates from Portuguese, Spanish, and Catalan. For And Other Stories she has translated from all three languages – from the Portuguese, *Now and at the Hour of Our Death* by Susana Moreira Marques, from the Catalan *Permafrost* by Eva Baltasar, and from the Spanish, *Slash and Burn* by Claudia Hernández, for which she won a PEN/Heim award. She has also translated works by Noemi Jaffe, Daniel Galera, and Geovani Martins, among others. She is a founding member of the Cedilla & Co. translators' collective, and currently lives in Providence, Rhode Island.